I HAVE CANCER?

Discussing the thoughts, feelings and emotions of a cancer diagnosis.

JOSHUA GLADDEN

First paperback edition: June 2023

Published by:
NarratusCreative | Narratus Press
P.O. Box 1413
Hamilton, OH 45012

Design: NarratusCreative | narratuscreative.com
Cover Photo Credits: Denise Chaney

Produced in the United States of America

DEDICATION

To my wife, Jamie: thank you for always being there for me. You have constantly supported me in everything I do, and I am so grateful. You have been with me from day one on my cancer journey. You have seen me at my best and my worst and you have loved me through it all. Even though we thought for a moment in our lives that "till death do us part" was coming sooner than we could have imagined, your love never wavered, and you have been with me though it all.
I love you.

TABLE OF CONTENTS

Introduction - 3

Chapter 1 – The Beginning - 7

Chapter 2 – Treatment - 19

Chapter 3 – What? - 29

Chapter 4 – Am I Going to Die? - 41

Chapter 5 – Why Me? - 51

Chapter 6 – What Did I Do to Deserve This? - 61

Chapter 7 – What about Jamie? - 73

Chapter 8 – Again? - 85

Chapter 9 – Dealing with Disappointment - 95

Chapter 10 – God in the Details - 107

Chapter 11 – Closing Thoughts -119

Introduction

CANCER. It's funny how one little word can mean so much. And even though it's just a word, it can have so much meaning to someone who hears it. Cancer may not mean much to you if it has never touched your life, but I can tell you first hand that when the doctor directs that little word to you, it *means* something. I remember when my doctor directed it towards me: panic set in, thoughts started racing through my brain and my emotions began to take over. I was in shock! You never think that something like that would happen to you, and when it does you can't believe it — and you definitely don't want to.

You have it. There is nothing you can do but sit there and think, *How did this happen? Why me? Are you sure?*

Even as those thoughts fill your head, you realize, it's true. The doctor was talking about you. *What's next? Am I going to die? What about my family? My job? My life?*

Clear thoughts start to come more easily, but where do you begin? It is funny how when we are faced with unthinkable news, our emotions seem to take over and questions pile up in our heads.

You know what? That's OK! It's a natural reaction. It is how we were created. Although we don't have all the answers — we want them, and we want them now!

It is crazy to think about, but who would have thought that such a small word could change the lives of millions of people? Honestly, cancer is not something that's even on our radar unless we have it or someone we care about is affected by it. It's funny how that works isn't it?

I know because I never thought about cancer until I was diagnosed with it. And in that moment I went through all of the emotions — and just like that, cancer meant more to me than anything else. It consumed my thoughts. Even though I tried to do a good acting job for everyone else, I couldn't hide from it. The thoughts and questions uncontrollably poured through my brain about what could, would and should happen.

Many of you too may have experienced this same feeling or you might have a close friend or family member that has heard those words. Maybe you're just wondering what all of this cancer stuff is about. I don't know why you decided to read this book, but my hope is that whoever you are and whatever your situation in relation to cancer is, that we can openly discuss the thoughts, feelings, and emotions that may accompany a cancer diagnosis and treatment.

I pray that I can be source of encouragement as I openly share and communicate my cancer story. My goal is not to teach, but rather have an open discussion of the many emotions that I myself, along with many others, have experienced throughout our personal cancer journeys.

No matter the diagnosis we can get through it. We can endure through the treatment and recovery and still live our lives with purpose. My personal experience with cancer and the treatments are all my own. Everyone will have their own personal cancer experiences and not one of them are the same. Some easier and some much worse, but hopefully this can be a starting point to understand some of the thoughts and emotions associated with those dreaded words: "You Have Cancer."

CHAPTER 1

The Beginning

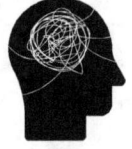

I was lying there on the bed, already prepped for surgery. My parents and my pastor had already been in to see me. My stepfather was the last person to come into the room to give me his version of the: "Everything's going to be OK," speech, when the doctor walked into the room. For the life of me, I have no idea why he decided five minutes before surgery to tell me what would change my life forever. With my wife and stepfather on ether side of the bed the doctor looked at us and said, "Well, I don't have to wait for the biopsy; I already know It's cancer."

"*What*?? How do you know?" My wife and I asked, almost in perfect harmony.

He replied, "The tumor markers in your blood work are high. When that happens I know It's cancer."

After that everything seems to be a blur. I remember my stepfather going to tell everyone the news, which began round two of people flooding into my little room. After the news I vaguely remember the anesthesiologist giving me more medicine to calm me down. Other than that, nothing. When you hear news like that it's almost like you're frozen in time. I can't think of a single thing anyone did or said from that moment until after surgery — but the thoughts in my head, I will never forget: *What? Am I going to die? Why me? What did I do to deserve this? What about Jamie?*

Unfortunately those words will never leave for some of us or maybe someone we know who has heard or will hear those words. I know they will never leave me: "You Have Cancer." That is not the exact phrase the doctor used while I was waiting for surgery, but I promise you that *IS* what I heard.

The unfortunate reality is that cancer is more common

today than it has ever been. The more unfortunate thing is that within the next few years it will be even more common than it is now. Researchers are continually trying to figure out cures and treatments to help keep cancer from coming back or spreading once it has been found, but what about the emotions and pain that's associated with it? That is something that no one except the person who has been diagnosed with the cancer can truly know and understand.

There are wonderful counselors and social workers that try to do their best to understand the feelings and emotions felt by someone who has been diagnosed with cancer, but the reality is that if you have never been affected by it personality it's just hard to understand what someone else is going through. It doesn't matter how much education, how many degrees, or the amount of schooling someone has if they have never been faced with the problems that you have faced; it's hard for them to truly understand what your dealing with. That seems to be evident in just about everyone that I've ever met.

If you have never been faced with divorce, sickness, pain, problems or even relationships that someone else has experienced, then you can never truly relate to their situation. No one wants advice from someone they feel can't relate to their situation. I understand that. And my personal experience with cancer is different than the one that you may be facing, but we do have some common ground in that we are both dealing with cancer.

My hope is that my personal experience can benefit you. Even though our experiences may not be the same, I do believe that most people diagnosed with this disease ask similar questions. More than likely we feel some of the same emotions. Some of you reading this may not be diagnosed with cancer and may not even know anyone who has, but hopefully my story can help you better understand the thoughts and emotions that can be associated with someone experiencing their cancer journey.

My Cancer Story

I guess to fully explain my cancer story I do need to start from the beginning. I began to notice that my testicle (I know, you probably weren't expecting that were you?) was getting larger than normal, but as any man would, I decided to "walk it off." What I mean is that I figured that I would give it some time and everything would be back to normal.

As time progressed there were no changes in my situation and to make things worse my wife kept telling me that I needed to go see the doctor. *Doctor*? *No way, who needs a doctor; give me a break it didn't hurt so why would I need to go to the doctor*? (Just a quick side note: now, more than ever do I realize why God created women, because men can be pretty stupid sometimes.) But honestly, what man wants to go to the doctor about "that area"? So I waited.

A few weeks passed and no change, well except that it may have gotten larger, so no positive change anyway. At this point I actually started to agree with my wife that I needed to go to the doctor, but I didn't let her know that. So like any guy trying not to let his wife know that she was right, I decided to do some research about what could be causing my problem. Well it didn't take long from a quick Google search to find out that nothing good could come from my little (or should I say, growing) problem. Even though I was secretly starting to get worried about my situation, my wife was a little more than aggravated with me and my stubbornness, so she made a phone call. Next thing I know I had a doctors appointment. Even though I was a little nervous about my condition I would have never have made the appointment to see the doctor about "that area", EVER!

That fateful Friday came. I used the excuse that I would be a little late for work because I had to take my wife to the doctor that morning. Now, I didn't lie about the doctor but I was so embarrassed by the location of my problem that I lied about *who* was going to the doctor. I guess I figured if there was no problem no one had to know my secret.

Anyway, I went to my primary care physician. I'm not sure if there is another word that could explain my extreme embarrassment — I was just plain embarrassed. That is exactly how I felt. I'll never forget it. I was filling out the paperwork for the doctors office, and as paperwork does, it kept prompting me to write down my problem and why I needed to see the doctor. I'm pretty sure that my face was glowing redder with every word that I wrote. There were a few other people in the waiting room as I sat there filling out the paperwork and I know that they probably could have cared less, but it felt as if they were all staring at me, laughing at my problem. I didn't think things could be worse until I realized that all of the receptionists and nurses sitting behind the counter were women. Oh how humiliating!

Finally, they called me back to be seen after what felt like an eternity. After a few quick questions and a brief look at the problem, my doctor referred me to a urologist. He suggested that time was of the essence because it could possibly be cancer. Wow, I wasn't expecting that! I was assuming that I had twisted it while I was playing outdoor games with the students at church and that everything would be back to normal within a reasonable amount of time. I guess, at the time, the reassuring thing in my mind was that my doctor, while firm on taking action immediately, didn't give me any reason to worry. I had no idea that my problem would end up being something as bad as it turned out to be. So taking his advice I let his receptionist make me an appointment with a urologist the next week (this time after I was off work).

I HAVE CANCER?

The next week came all too soon. I found myself sitting in the waiting room of the second doctor within only a few days of the first. Considering that I hadn't been to see a doctor since my last physical for sports my sophomore year in high school, this was all a little much for me.

Once again, what felt like an eternity passed before I was called back to see the urologist. And again, I had to face the embarrassment of someone besides my wife looking at my private area. This time, the doctor wasn't just looking, but also had to touch and feel and move and... Well you get the point. It was horrible. During this visit the doctor decided to take an ultrasound of my testicle — yeah, I thought they were only for pregnant women too — obviously not.

After all of the tests, he told me he wanted to get another ultrasound from the hospital so that he could get more extensive data than his machine could provide. *OK*, I was thinking, *not so bad*. I could deal with all of that until he told me what no man ever expects to hear in his life: I was going to have surgery to remove my testicle!

Who? ...What? ... When? ... Where? ... and ... Why?

Those were all valid questions at this point. His answer wasn't something that I was excited about either. The reason he would have to remove the testicle was because it possibly could be cancer. He was not saying for sure that it was, but there was a chance. Honestly, that didn't bother me that much because I was sure of the fact that I wouldn't have cancer. Besides, I was completely healthy. I had never been sick except the occasional bug that some over the counter medicine took care of in about 48 hours. So, no I wasn't all that concerned about the cancer. What didn't sit well with me is that I was going to lose something that no man wants to lose. A small, side-note that I should mention: I had only been married for a little over a year. So his quick decision of wanting to take away a part of my body that I had just begun to enjoy wasn't sitting so well with me.

Trying to digest all of the information that I had just received didn't come so easily either. Needless to say after a lot of talking and deep discussion with my wife, we decided that if the procedure had to be done, well we just had to do it.

I did go to the hospital for my ultrasound the next day. I wasn't feeling nearly as nervous or embarrassed since this was going to be the third time in almost as many days of letting a stranger see my private parts... Until I ran into a good friend's wife at the hospital. It wasn't the running into her that was bad, it was the realization that she was in her scrubs — she worked there. She was a radiologist technician. That's what scared me. What I didn't know until later was that a radiologist tech doesn't perform that test I was receiving and she didn't even work in that department. Oh, what I would have given to hide during the time I spent waiting to be called back for my test, after seeing her.

Although relieved once I was called back and found out that she wouldn't be doing the test, it still wasn't perfect. Up until now my doctors had been men, but not for this. The lady doing the test was about my age and very nice and very professional. Probably noticing my embarrassment, she kept the conversation going throughout the procedure, but I was less than comfortable. Sitting in a room with nothing between your manhood while being probed by another woman that's not your wife — I must admit, I would have rather have been hit by a semi-truck, then backed over and hit again than to have been in that room at that very moment. What felt as if another eternity had finally passed, I was still alive. Nothing was hurt other than my pride three times over. Now I had to face the urologist again.

My next couple of visits to the urologist were not nearly as bad, only because my wife and parents met me there and gave me good moral support. Since my wife and I were so confused and in such a daze with the whole situation, my parents were a huge blessing by helping us ask the questions that needed to be asked. After only a couple visits to the urologist we went ahead and scheduled the surgery.

So begins my cancer story. After the surgery my doctor assured me that everything was out that needed to be out and that after I was healed up from the surgery we would begin the next steps of cancer prevention.

Two weeks after my operation I went to have the staples closing my incision removed and I found out a little about my tumor. It was considered a non-seminomatous tumor. It was an 80% embryonal, germ cell tumor and the other 20% was a yolk sack tumor. I still don't completely understand the terminology but I do know that the 80% was the cancerous part. We also were able to catch the cancer before it got any worse or spread elsewhere in my body.

The unfortunate part is that it was a very fast acting cancer and there was no time to waist in preventive treatment. Since my testicle was removed, there was now no host home for the cancer. But if there was any cancer left that the urologist missed, it could spread throughout my body very quickly. Because of that decisions had to be made relatively fast.

After my operation I was sent to get my first of many CT scans. The purpose of these scans was to make sure that the cancer had not spread throughout my body. The doctor gave me two choices on preventive treatment: Choice A was observation, consisting of CT scans every two months, which would be bad on my body because of the excessive radiation that I would be receiving or Choice B was to have a lymphadectomy which is a surgery that would remove the lymph nodes on the left side of my body. Most doctors at that time who preformed the surgery only averaged one or two a year. As you can tell, it wasn't a very common surgery. Along with that, the side effects were not too promising. Honestly, there are too many to list, but the one that scared me the most had the potential for me to never be able to ejaculate again. (Remember, I had only been married for a little over a year at this point — that didn't sound good at all!)

As my wife, Jamie, and I began to look over the positives and negatives of both options we decided against the lymph node surgery and to just go with the observation method. Needless to say it wasn't the easiest choice to make and definitely not the most popular choice by her parents or mine, but the second choice was non-negotiable for us.

At last it was decision day. Along with my wife, I wanted my parents to come along to ask any questions that Jamie or I may not have thought about, so off we went. What we didn't know at the time was that this would be the last time I would see that urologist. I was called back to see the doctor and believe it or not, as we were all in the room waiting for the doctor to come in, the fire alarm went off. I know it sounds crazy but we all had to exit the building and wait outside to see if the building would burn away only to find out a child had pulled the fire alarm.

On a day you have to make a decision that could mean life or death it wasn't what I wanted to happen to say the least. A nurse came out to get us and we all went back inside and continued to wait for the doctor. He arrived shortly after the alarm episode. When we began to talk about my procedure and the cancer, he finally asked Jamie and me what we had decided: observation, surgery or chemotherapy?

What? *A third choice*? I could have jumped out of my seat and punched him in the face, except for my newfound curiosity about this third choice. He had never mentioned a third choice before. I don't know if he had forgotten or if he just really wanted to do the surgery, but this was the first time I had heard of this "third choice".

Since the first two options weren't to my liking, I was excited to find out about this third choice. My urologist's office made an appointment for me to see an oncologist about the possibility of chemotherapy. I was excited, yet very nervous about the option of chemotherapy because of all of the things that I had heard about it. However, I had to at least go see what it was all about.

Jamie had to work and couldn't come with me to my appointment, so my mother went with me to talk about the possibilities with the oncologist. As the doctor walked into the room, even though we had never met, somehow I immediately felt better. I don't really know how or why but as she began to speak it felt as if a burden was being lifted off of my shoulders. As we began to go over my diagnosis and the reason I was seeing her, little by little I began to feel so much better about my situation. By the end of our conversation I was ready to do anything she said. I guess it helped that she had just gotten back from a huge oncologists meeting in which she was the keynote speaker on testicular cancer. Or it may have been what she said during that meeting about the lymphadectomy. It had been discussed and was found to be completely ineffective in cancer prevention.

Honestly, it was everything from her knowledge to her understanding of my situation, all the way from the way she presented herself. If I can borrow the famous line from the now classic movie "Jerry Maguire", she "had me at hello". Chemotherapy was the option for me. I now had a new doctor a new hope, and there is absolutely no doubt in my mind that God directed me to her. I still remember that afternoon, after my mother and I left the office. We looked at one another and agreed that chemotherapy was the right decision for me.

I understand that there are several ways to treat cancer and some types require different treatments. In no way am I trying to advertise for chemotherapy above other options, but in my situation, it worked for me. Let me say this: I definitely don't want to make light of the chemotherapy treatment process. I would not wish that on anyone.

As we continue, I will elaborate more on my chemotherapy treatments and the feelings associated with them, but hopefully as I have been able to share the beginnings of my cancer experience, you will have noticed how quickly things happen. From the day my wife made my first doctors appointment (end of May 2008) to my first day of chemotherapy (first week of July 2008) was only a little over one month. A month may seem like a long time but believe me it's not long enough.

That has to be one of the hardest things about being diagnosed with cancer; you must make life-long, life-changing and life-saving decisions in a matter of days.

Thankfully, I had a wonderful support group of family and church friends that were able to help Jamie and myself throughout our decision making process. But, as you can imagine, even with such a great support base around me it wasn't all easy. There were many sleepless nights as questions, concerns, and worries filled my head. As we continue into my story I hope to show you that even in uncertain times we can still find hope in our situation.

CHAPTER 2

Treatment

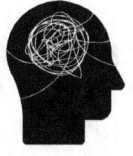

The decision was over. My lymph nodes were staying inside my body; and even though observation was still apart of my new treatment plan, it wasn't the only part. Chemotherapy here I come. I must say that even though I was feeling better about actually having a plan and I felt really good about my new doctor, I was still nervous. I had heard about chemo before, but didn't know too much about it...well, I didn't know anything about it except you lose your hair. So, I was going to be learning as I went through the process.

As I said before, I was extremely impressed by my oncologist. Her demeanor, her knowledge and her personality were all great. I felt as if she really cared for me as a person, not just a patient. I think that was the most important part of feeling good about my decision to opt for the chemotherapy route. I don't know if you are familiar with chemotherapy, but basically it is an IV drug that uses chemicals to kill off fast growing cells in the body. Since cancer cells grow at a faster rate than others, it is an effective way to get rid of them quickly. There are several types of chemo drugs that are used depending on many different factors of the patient and the particular cancer being treated. For me, my chemo regimen consisted of three different types of drugs: Bleomycin, Etoposide and Cisplatin.

I'm glad I initially felt good about choosing to go the chemo route because if I didn't, I don't know if I could have made it through the treatments. It was horrible! I understand that not all treatments are the same, but for me it was bad. I guess it should have been expected. When we were going over the treatment plan and regimen, the oncologist, looked at my wife and me and told us, "I'm going to give you an aggressive chemo treatment. I'm going to put you to the point of death, but because you are young and healthy — other than the cancer — you will be fine."

Huh? *To the point of death*? *Did I just hear that correctly*? Wow, that was unexpected! But, believe me when I say, she wasn't lying. Treatments were hard, really hard. It was one of those, "I wouldn't wish that on anyone, ever," kind of hard.

The reason for her "aggressive" treatment plan was two-fold: First, the particular type of cancer I had was considered an aggressive, fast moving and fast growing cancer. Because of that she wanted to treat it hard and fast. Secondly, because I was young and otherwise healthy, my body could endure a heavy dosage of the chemotherapy drugs and the longer you are taking chemo the worse it can be for your body. So from my understanding I had one of the largest dosages of chemo treatments available at that time.

The way it worked out was that I went for treatments five straight days, Monday through Friday, and had the weekend off. I went back the following Monday and then had the rest of that week off. The next Monday I started another week-long cycle, off the weekend and went back the following Monday for my last treatment. In total my treatment only lasted for 12 days but like I said, it was a very aggressive, hard and fast type of treatment. Although it may not have lasted several months like you may have heard or experienced, I can tell you first hand that it felt longer than two week plus one day of treatments.

On the weekend after each week-long cycle and for about a week after I was done receiving my chemo treatments I had to give myself a Leukine injection in my stomach. This shot was to help produce white blood cells in my body, which fight infection and sickness, because the chemo weakens the immune system. You are a lot more susceptible to viruses and sickness when taking chemotherapy so you have to take precautions. You self-isolate to avoid getting sick during chemotherapy and even for a while after your treatments are done.

I don't want to jump around too much, but I do want to explain the process I went through for each chemo treatment, especially if you are unfamiliar with how it works. It has been several years ago now, so the process may have changed a bit and it could vary from doctor to doctor.

For me, when I arrived at the office, it was just like any other doctor's visit. I would sign in and wait to be called back. The weirdest part of the waiting room, both during my treatment time or even when I would come back for my normal "check-up" visits, were all of the people staring at me. This time is was true. It wasn't that I *felt* they were staring at me out of my embarrassment — they really were staring at me. I could even hear some of them occasionally whispering about me too. I knew what it was about though; I was really young. I was only 24 at the time and I looked even younger. Most of the people being seen at the "cancer doctor" are, as you can imagine, older. I would say that 95% of the patients were my grandparents' age, the rest were my parents' age or a little older, and then there was me. So, needless to say, I stuck out from the crowd.

After sitting through the awkwardness of the waiting room, I would be called back and escorted to the phlebotomy room. There I would get hooked up to my IV, either injected into my arm or flushed out if it was being reused.

Many people who receive chemotherapy, blood transfusions or regularly get IV injections have ports. These ports are surgically placed, typically in the top part of your chest so that whether the phlebotomists are taking blood or giving the patient an IV, they can do this through the port instead of having to get a new stick each time. The port allows for easy access to the patient's veins, especially if it is needed for a prolonged period of time. This way, the patient is only being poked by the needle once rather than the possibility of multiple sticks trying to find a well-used and possibly blown vein. Ports are widely used in chemotherapy patients because the veins are harder to access while receiving treatments. Chemo can make veins smaller and harder which makes it difficult and painful to find a good vein, which is why many people choose to utilize a port when going through treatments. .

Even though I could have gotten a port, I did not. My treatment plan was super aggressive and would be done in such a short period of time that I didn't need it, so they used the traditional IV method. They were able to reuse my IV twice during each week-long cycle so that I didn't have to get a new one every day, which was nice. The nurses would just wrap it up after my treatment. The next day, they used a flush to clean it out so that it could be used again for treatments that day.

But, after a day or so, the pain with each new IV inserted into my arm was immense. I remember telling my wife that it felt like they were trying to put a McDonalds® straw into my vein. Like I said earlier, after a while the chemo will destroy your veins making it harder for them to be used. To this day I still have trouble on occasion trying to give blood out of my left arm, which was used primarily for my treatments.

Before I move on from the phlebotomy room I have a funny little story... Well it's funny now. At the time it wasn't so funny, especially for my Dad.

On this particular day — it was probably my 3rd or 4th day of that week-long cycle — my dad had driven me to my chemo appointment. There was no way I could have driven myself. I was too weak. Dad walked back into the phlebotomy waiting area with me and from his seat, he could see me getting my IV inserted. That day I had to get a new IV installed. I was extremely weak and very nauseous. I had been prescribed an anti-nausea medication that I had to carry with me and I needed it that day because I was feeling light headed. The lady who was changing out my IV asked if I had it with me, and I did. I leaned down from my seat to get it out of my bag as she was saying, "Stop!" But it was too late.

I don't remember anything after that except the back of my head pounding as I looked up at my Dad and the phlebotomist, who were both calling my name and asking me if I was okay. I had passed out — apparently hard. My Dad told me later that he thought I had died. He was watching me and he said that as I started to lean down, in my extremely weakened state, my eyes rolled to the back of my head, my body convulsed and I flew backwards, hitting my head on the wall behind me. I don't know how long I was out. I assume that it was my Dad's parental nervousness that made him think I had died; but the phlebotomist, who I developed a good relationship with over our time together, was seemingly rattled as well. So much so that she came into the chemo room a couple of times that day to check on me and she made sure that my doctor and nurses knew what was going on before I was allowed to receive my treatment for the day. I told you — crazy story, huh?

Anyway, after the trip to the phlebotomy room was over and my IV was either installed or flushed, I was taken back to the chemo room. That's a room I'll never forget. The first thing I noticed every time I walked into that big open space was the smell. I can't describe it. I don't know if it was a cleaner that was used or the plastic IV bags full of drugs, but whatever it was, that distinct smell punched you right in the face as you entered the room. Even now if I detect a whiff of whatever that was, it takes me back to that room and I will always associate that scent with chemo. I know it sounds crazy but to me that's what chemo smells like. Yuck!

As I would enter the chemo room there was a nurses station on the left side and the rest of the room was filled with those hospital grade recliners. You know the ones that are a chair — only the sense of the word, chair — tall, stiff, blue, vinyl covered recliners. Behind each row of recliners was a small wall separating the back of each row of "recliners" from the others. Sitting on the tops of the walls were boxes of tissues and jars full of Jolly Ranchers®. One of the side effects while receiving chemo treatments is that your mouth gets really dry, so the Jolly Ranchers® were there to help keep it from becoming unbearable. I went through a ton of them during my treatments so it makes me nauseous just talking about them, even right now. After picking out my chair for the day and getting situated in it, the chemo bag was attached and the fun would begin.

I have heard that radiation treatments can actually hurt as you are receiving them, but that isn't the case with chemo. You don't even feel it. If you have ever been given an IV bag of anything you know that you can't feel the liquid as it enters your veins. It is the same with the chemotherapy treatment, you can't feel anything, but it makes you extremely tired and weak. And, at least for me, the treatments made me feel like I was dying.

My mom was telling me recently how she remembered that I told her I just wanted to die after the second day of treatment. I don't remember saying that to her, but I believe it because I remember feeling that way. She said that after I told her that she just looked at me and told me to sleep, because I couldn't feel the pain and weakness in my body if I was asleep. She was right. Most people are sleeping throughout the duration of their treatments so I followed suit. By the time you have all of those chemicals literally running through your veins, there isn't much more you can do other than to sleep. I remember having great aspirations of reading and listening to music. I even carried a bag with a book, some magazines and my iPhone for music, but rarely did I ever do any of those things. I spent most of my time asleep, but even if I wasn't sleeping I was too tired and weak to even pull out a book or my phone. I just sat in silence, as each drip made its way down the tube and into my arm.

As I said earlier, I was given a large dosage of medicine. Because of that I was typically the first or one of the first patients of the day to enter the chemo room as well as the last or one of the last to leave that afternoon. Depending on the day my treatments would last from 4 ½ to 5 ½ hours. As you can imagine that makes for a long day, just waiting for your IV bags to empty out.

You know, it's funny, but as I look back at my treatment time, it doesn't seem so bad now — but it was. The way it made me feel, the lack of energy and the total body weakness was horrible! On the positive side, there wasn't much physical pain associated with the treatment plan or process, but being so weak and helpless made it miserable. Honestly, that is what made the treatments so bad for me — not being able to do anything for myself. I was just too weak. It's hard to explain, physical pain wasn't really there but it was the mental defeat that played the largest part. What I mean is that my body was so weak, I could not function. Everything I tried to do was a chore. Walking to the toilet almost couldn't happen. I lived my life for those couple of weeks on the couch or in the bed and that was it. There wasn't anything else I could do. It was so strenuous to get back and forth to the bathroom or even more, to take a shower. Because of this my wife, Jamie, had to lift me in and out of the bathtub so she could bath me as I sat in the tub pretty much helpless. After she washed me, she would have to dry me off, help me into my clothes and basically help me walk to the bed. I tried to be as independent as I could, but those simple things that even now I take for granted, I couldn't do without her help.

That's the mental defeat I was dealing with. I am an extremely independent person and hate asking for help for anything, yet there I was in need of help just to survive. There were some times when I was so tired and weak that I couldn't even feed myself. Jamie would have to help me with that as well. That was very humbling for me and I hated every minute of it. Being so physically weak and tired, I would often become brash even lashing out in aggravation and anger. Not on purpose, it just happened. So much so that Jamie told me I wouldn't have to worry about cancer killing me because she would take care of me first! Yikes! Luckily, several years later, and still counting, she hasn't acted on that threat just yet.

I understand that not everyone will have the same type of cancer that I had and that there are various different experiences with cancer treatment, but the biggest thing for me was to overcome the aggravation that I couldn't do what I wanted to do or what I normally could do. It was terrible to have my mind functioning 100%, yet not being able to physically do anything. Because of that, small things would seem to get on my nerves — things that normally would never bother me at all. Unfortunately, I didn't know how to handle those feelings at the time and came off brash and angry — mostly to my wife. It's amazing how quickly I let my physical incapabilities overtake my mental state and in turn, my attitude and actions, but I did. For me that was by far the most difficult part of my treatment.

CHAPTER 3

What?

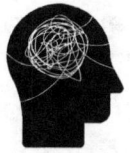

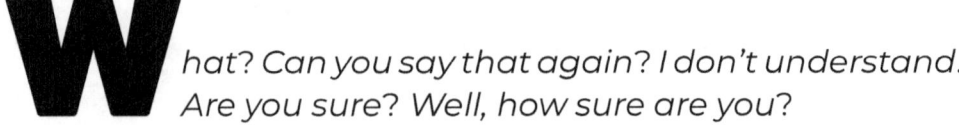

hat? Can you say that again? I don't understand. Are you sure? Well, how sure are you?

If you have ever been told that you have cancer I'm pretty sure that you, like me, had thoughts like these running through your head too. I'm not sure if I actually verbalized any of those questions out loud, but I know it was what I was thinking in the moment. Questions arise so fast you don't know what to do and no matter how hard you try to ask all of the things that are spinning through your head, you never can seem to get them out.

That's the feeling in that moment. Time seems to stand still the second you hear the news. A million thoughts arise while your throat starts to close and your mind goes into overdrive. Finally, when you can muster up enough energy to ask a question, through the emotions of the moment, it never seems to be the one you really wanted to ask. For me that seemed to happen every single time I walked into the doctor's office. I was always prepared to get every question I had thought of answered. But, I never did. It seemed like after every visit, not only did I not get all of my questions answered, but I walked away with what seemed to be a thousand more. I needed those questions answered.

Through all of the hustle and bustle of life we never seem to be fully prepared when unexpected moments arise. The truth is, even if we had just the right amount of time to prepare and even when we're not taken by surprise, it seems we are never truly prepared. A deadline at work, picking up the kids, even trying to get somewhere on time, it never seems we have enough time.

When we first got married, I thought my wife was one of the worst people in the world about being on time to do anything. Years later I have realized that she isn't as bad as I once thought. In my defense, at that time I was "Mr. Punctual". If I was supposed to be somewhere at a specific time, I was there 15 minutes beforehand. I used to be the guy that if it took an hour to get somewhere, I would leave two hours early, just to make sure I knew exactly where I was going. Then I may have proceeded to drive around or wait in the car until I could arrive my usual 15 minutes early. As you can imagine, in the early stages of our marriage, we had a few disagreements on time management. Jamie would often tell me that even though I may leave early I couldn't control everything, like the traffic or a flat tire and believe it or not— the world wouldn't end if I wasn't right on time or even early for something! The audacity!

Not only am I, "Mr. Punctual", but I'm also a guy who is very set in my ways. I have my own routine for doing just about everything. I must admit my wife has helped me make changes in that area too, but overall I am still a very routine person. I have a routine for just about everything I do, everyday. I wash my hands first thing when I get into the shower, followed by washing my hair. I must do that before I wash my face and so on. I brush my teeth the same way each time... I'm sure you get the picture. I like my routines.

Since I am such a "routined" person I know that I handle new things a little differently than most, especially my wife. If something changes in her day she just goes with it, having no worries. She adjusts and moves on with life. I envy that quality in her since I am just about the complete opposite in just about every way. If something happens unexpectedly in my routine I must think about what happened, and then proceed by thinking how I am going to deal with it. After thinking about it, I continue to think about it some more before I can continue with my day. I can't completely understand the way Jamie operates and I know she doesn't understand my way of doing things either, but that's okay. I think that is probably what keeps our marriage going. I know it keeps it interesting!

You may be like me — always prepared or slightly over-prepared, or you may be more like my wife and just "go with the flow". I like how Dave Ramsey describes the differences in people through their finances. He puts them into two categories the "nerds" and the "free spirits". I'll give you one guess which one I am compared to my wife. That's right, I'm the nerd and I'm okay with that!

Whatever the case may be there are just some instances where we can't control anything. Situations where the over prepared nerd, in all of our efforts, can't figure out where we messed up. And even the free-spirits have circumstances where they can't seem to grasp the situation fast enough to just "go with the flow". No matter how prepared or how easily we can adjust, there are some things that happen in life that no one can really prepare for, understand or fix. That's the thing about cancer that I don't think any of us can truly understand. Question after question, book after book, there are no real answers that make us feel that we can really understand what is going on.

I am the type of person who looks at something in depth. Even though it may take some time by doing the right research and talking with the right people, I can normally figure out a solution to just about any problem I might be having (it may not always be right, but we won't get into that). I know that cancer doesn't automatically mean certain death or that you will become some sort of test subject who can never have a normal life. No, it's not like that at all. Even so, those things do seem to creep into your thinking.

So at each doctor's visit we learned to ask every question we could think of only to get more information we had to process. This I know all too well as do so many other people out there who have been diagnosed with cancer. The greatest advice that I can give someone about asking questions about their cancer is this: *No matter how many questions we can ask or how many articles or books we read, we will never seem to find the answer that really satisfies us, so find peace within yourself with the answers you find.* When you can find peace in your situation, is when you can move on with your life. Don't let the unknown dictate your life, take hold of it and keep moving forward!

When I was told that I had cancer I had so many questions about how I got it and why I had it. I imagine I'm just like anyone else who has ever heard those words. The questions arise quickly. "What?" is one question that will follow almost every explanation that you hear or find in your research. I know it was that way with me.

Before each doctor's appointment I began to get prepared and I was not alone in my question making. My wife and parents were a part of the process, so the day before an appointment, we compiled a list of extensive questions so that I was primed and ready to ask every question in my arsenal. Yet, as prepared as I was my inquiries never seemed to get completely answered. At least not to my liking. Even in all of my over-preparedness, my organization, my punctuality or routine, the questions I had could never be answered 100%.

Because with every appointment and every conversation more and more questions arose. What is funny about all of these questions is that for every one that I could think up someone else would bring up another point. That point would then lead to a whole new series of questions. I can't begin to tell you about all of the questions my family and friends would ask that either that I hadn't thought about or that I just had no answer for. Day after day, thought after thought, question after question seemed to build yet I never seemed to be able to find any peace in the answers that I found.

That is the one thing that I hated most about each appointment; more questions *after* the visit than before. You may be thinking that with all of the technology we have access to today, all of my questions should have answers and you may be right. Yet, in all honesty, not all of the answers are things you want to hear.

If I can give some advice about question asking, most of the time it is better to not try and find the answers yourself and just listen to your doctor(s). Now, I'm not saying to just be ignorant or to be a "yes" man or woman. If I would have listened to certain things one of my doctors had suggested, I may not be here or at least I would not have they quality of life that I have today.

What I am saying is that sometimes the Internet and books are wrong, or at least one sided. They can't answer every question and about every person or situation either.

It goes back to finding that peace within yourself through your situation. It may help you understand what I am trying to convey by using an illustration. Let's use skydiving as our example.

I have never been skydiving nor have I ever had the desire to do so. Nevertheless, if I was going to go skydiving, I'm not going without a parachute. That makes sense, right? So, if one day I decided to go skydiving, I would begin to research the different businesses that specialize in skydiving. Then, I would look up the statistics of how many dives each company has done and their success rate, making sure that the instructors were registered and licensed to skydive.

After that, I would visit the place and check it out for myself. I would then have a basic knowledge of what skydiving is and how to do it, but I still wouldn't know everything about it or even be an expert on the subject.

That's how I see being diagnosed with cancer. No matter how much research about it or how many questions we ask, we can't know everything about it. When we're diagnosed, we have such a small window of time before we have to start making decisions. We are definitely not going to become experts in that time frame.

Back to my skydiving analogy, let's that after my research I decided to go skydiving at ABC Skydiving Company. I'm all suited up and ready to go, but when we we're going over the final instructions, I don't fully understand something that the instructor was saying. Would it be wise to just not say anything? No, of course not! If I don't understand something I'm going to ask questions. If I still don't understand I'm going to ask more questions, or perhaps go to a different skydiving company that can help me fully understand what I am doing before taking the plunge at 10,000 feet.

I feel strongly about this with a cancer diagnosis and treatment. It's okay to ask questions and if you still don't understand or don't feel good about them – keep on asking. If that doesn't seem to help, go somewhere else and get a second opinion. Ultimately you have to feel good about what's going on.

We all understand that if our skydiving instructor said we didn't need to use the parachute, we are gong to start asking a lot of rapid-fire questions and we are going somewhere else if our questions aren't answered to our satisfaction.

I wish it were that easy about getting answers from our doctors, but unfortunately it's not. I guess the thing to know about getting answers to your questions is that you just have to learn to become comfortable with the answers that you get. There has to be some sort of trust between you and your physician. If you know that they are the best person for you then you may just have to trust them, even if you don't completely understand all of the facts. They are the doctors; we are not.

Even as I say that, I would also caution that it is okay to not settle on the first physician you see or even the one that the insurance company suggests. It's okay to question their opinions and motives. It's okay to feel them out and see where they stand on issues that are important to your personal health choices.

Being completely transparent, I didn't feel good about my urologist and honestly still to this day believe that he didn't tell me about chemotherapy because he wanted to perform that surgery on me. Because of that I am so glad that I didn't just jump on board with what he was suggesting, even pushing me towards.

I believe this in every aspect of your personal health too. This is your body. These are your decisions. Don't feel trapped! It's terrible that you or a loved one has to make these decisions, so make sure that when you do make them, you are comfortable about your treatment and your care. We may not get all the answers we want or even understand everything like we wish we could but eventually we must place our trust in someone else. This can be difficult. Decisions must be made and we have to trust that God has led us to the people who know more about our situation than we do.

Once I realized that, it seemed to make things a little easier. After I found my oncologist and realized that she knew more about my condition than I did, my questions seemed to slowly disappear. Now I'm not saying that will happen for everyone, nor should it, but after I was able to come to the realization that neither I or nor anyone else I knew understood my cancer like my doctor, it just got easier to trust her. She knew what she was doing and everything would be fine. I give credit to my doctor but the real reason I was able to find peace in my unanswered questions was through my relationship with God.

Constant prayer, asking Him to lead me to the right doctors and to give me peace throughout these decisions was how I was able to find my peace. It sounds stereotypical to say but I am sure that God lead me to my doctor. From the moment I met her I had a peace about my situation. Once He led me to my oncologist and through prayer, I began to lose my worry and gain my peace through Him.

Another thing that I believe the Lord led me to do during this time was to stop feeding my emotions. Sounds crazy, I know. What is *feeding my emotions* anyway? For me not feeding my emotions meant that I had to stop listening to what the world said about cancer. I stopped reading articles on the Internet and asked my family and friends not to talk about what they thought I needed or should do. I understood that they were just worried about me and wanted to pass along any information that they received, but I believe sometimes it is best not to know. Some of the information that is "found" may not even be true anyway.

I know what you may be thinking. Here I have been telling you to ask questions and to research your diagnosis, and now I'm saying it may be best not to know. I'm not trying to speak out of both sides of my mouth here. I do believe it is important to ask questions and gather information so that you can be informed. But, I also believe that if we are not careful, in all of our research, study and questioning we can get overwhelmed and frustrated by not finding the answers we want. When we get to that point it may be best to just stop. The old adage, "ignorance is bliss", well, it may bear truthful in this situation.

Again, I'm not trying to be difficult to understand, but sometimes the less you "know" about something the better, because that way you can't worry about it!

There are some people in this world that, every time a new virus or sickness hits the news, they suddenly have it (I know a few of these people, as I'm sure you do too). I've even known people who won't go outside or visit certain places after they have heard of a virus or disease that has popped up. Should we be cautious? Yes. Should we let these things dictate our lives? No.

The comedian Jeff Foxworthy tells a joke about his wife that I think is absolutely hilarious, partly because of the type of cancer I had. The joke goes something like this: He said that his wife was always watching television shows that identified different diseases and their symptoms. By end of each episode, after his wife heard the laundry list of symptoms highlighted, she would be suffering with the disease the show was featuring. Mr. Foxworthy said that one night as they were watching the TV show, his wife began saying, "Oh No! I have all of the symptoms!" It was at that point he had to stop her and tell her that she in fact did not have testicular cancer, nor did she even have "testiculars". I know that it's just a joke, but you see, if his wife hadn't ever watched that television show she would have never worried about having some sort of sickness.

Again, I am not condoning being ignorant of the fact that we are sick and need help, but I do believe we worry ourselves with things that don't even need to be worried about. In my case, I decided that it would be in my best interest to stop listening to or reading what other people's opinions were of my situation, but rather to trust that God would give wisdom to my doctor to properly care for me. Often we can get trapped into thinking, saying or doing something out of the fear, either from our circumstances or from the unknown. The best way to stop being afraid is to stop feeding our fear.

When we are facing many of the "What?" questions in our lives, lets make sure that we don't let them overload our thoughts and actions. It is so easy to say, but so hard to do. When confronted by circumstances over which we have no control, we must always remember that as much as we try to seek for answers, we will always have unanswered questions.

For every question that I asked my doctors, I would always walk away with more. Even though they tried to explain and gave me adequate time to ask my questions, every time I got into my car to go home I remembered more and more questions that I just forgot to ask. Sometimes it was due to the fact that I didn't want to waste any more of the doctor's time and other times I realized that I would lose my train of thought as my brain tried to grasp everything being explained, so I would forget what my next question even was.

Whatever the case may be, I know that even as prepped and prepared I was for each visit to the doctor, I was continually unprepared for what was to come. We must be able to come to a place where we can put our faith in our God, and let Him direct our path. In doing that we can find peace in all of our "What?" questions that arise.

CHAPTER 4

Am I Going to Die?

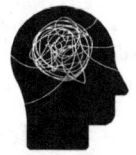

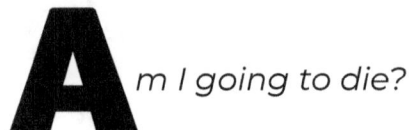**A**m I going to die?

That's the one question I believe everyone diagnosed with cancer asks. I don't understand how one word can have so much negativity associated with it, but it does. Just hearing it somehow gives you that spine tingling uneasy feeling: Cancer.

There is not another word that once heard is immediately associated with death. I don't know what it is about death that scares us. Maybe it's the fear of the unknown or it could be the anticipated pain we associate with death. Could it be the heartache of leaving a loved one, or the thought of how you will die? Whatever the case, it seems to be universal. The thought of death makes us afraid. No one wants to die in a fire or have some slow and painful death from a sickness or disease. Honestly, people would much rather die painlessly in their sleep, after they have lived a good long life. Unfortunately, we don't get to decide how or even when that time will be. That is left up to our Creator.

Recently I was reminded of this as I was driving. I noticed an SUV that had run off the side of the road. It was laying on its passenger side, wheels still spinning, smoke coming from the hood. I was one of the first people to see it. I pulled over to make sure whoever was involved was alright and out of the vehicle, because it looked like it may catch fire. Two other men got to the vehicle before I did and were already in action trying to get the unconscious driver out of his SUV. The back hatch was jammed and couldn't be opened, so the only way for us to get the man out of the vehicle was through the drivers side door, which was pointing towards the sky.

With a lot of effort we soon found out that there was no way to get the man out without the help of the fire department. Both of the other men had dropped down inside the car, trying to hold the unconscious man up to allow him to keep breathing. I was standing on top of the turned over vehicle holding the driver's door open so that the two men had room in the cramped space. Once the fire department arrived they had to use the "jaws of life" in order to remove the roof of the SUV and get the driver safely out. Unfortunately, as the emergency crew worked on removing the roof, the driver passed away in the arms of one of the men who had been trying to get him out.

After the man was removed and examined, it was thought that a medical event, possibly a heart attack or a stroke, had caused him to run off of the road. Once the police had gotten their reports, I got into my car to drive away from the sight of the accident and I was reminded of Solomon's words in the book of Ecclesiastes.

In chapter three he starts off by saying, "There is a time for everything, a season for every activity under heaven. A time to be born and a time to die..." (Ecclesiastes 3: 1-2a NLT)

There is a time to die. I don't know when that is, but for that man on that February afternoon, his season here on earth ended. I couldn't help but wonder about his eternal destination. *Was he a Believer?* I felt sorry for his family who would have to be located and then told the terrible news. And then I thought about his day: when he woke up that morning or even as he was driving down the road that afternoon, he didn't know he wouldn't make it to the end of that day – he didn't even make it to his destination. We are not promised tomorrow, cancer or not.

The thought of death can be scary, but we cannot let our fear dictate our lives. Cancer doesn't always mean death, so we shouldn't live in fear of something that isn't a certainty. I can honestly say that even though I thought of the possibility of death upon the news of my cancer, I was never fearful of it. The only reason I know that I was not fearful of death is because of the certainty of my eternity through my relationship with Jesus Christ. I know that when I die here on earth, I will begin my new eternal life with God. It is only because of this that throughout my diagnosis and cancer treatment, I never feared death. I can't really explain the calm; it was something indescribable. Peace in a time of turmoil. I can't fully wrap my head around it, but I know it was God.

Well, you may be wondering – *how can you not fear death*? That is a logical question and what I just shared is true — it was only through my relationship with Jesus that I was able to navigate such an uncertain time in my life. However, I wasn't completely fearless about death. I just wasn't afraid of dying. *What*?? I know, I know. That doesn't make any sense at all does it?

I guess I can try to explain it like this: the fear of dying or even the pain associated with it didn't bother me. Honestly, I know this may be hard to believe, but the actual death thing didn't bother me. The thing that I had to deal with wasn't if or when I was going to die, but rather leaving behind the people who are so important to me. I almost couldn't bear the fact that barely into a year of marriage and I could possibly be leaving my wife a widow.

Even as I write those words it still unnerves me a little. This was by far the thing that scared me the most about my cancer, not death, but leaving the love of my life alone. That is what got me. She probably doesn't need me nearly as much as I need her, but man, I just couldn't hardly think about it without getting emotional. Leaving behind family and friends, knowing that you won't be around for any more holidays, anniversaries, birthdays or whatever else, is a tough pill to swallow, but, leaving my wife – that hurt! Being so young at the time, I was 24, and being newly married, it was excruciating to consider.

At that time, Jamie and I didn't even want children, but even now, years later thinking about our son, Jonathan – I can't fathom! Leaving my son fatherless, probably would have been the hardest thing, even harder than leaving my wife. I'm sure of it. That would have been my greatest fear in death – leaving my son behind!

Even though I wasn't truly fearful, I knew the likelihood of death was closer than ever before in my life and there was nothing that I or anyone else could do about it. The only thing I could do and try to control was me. I tried to be strong for my wife, my parents, my family and my friends. I'm not sure that I did a good job at it, but what else was I supposed to do?

There is no real answer as to how you handle the stress and grief when faced with what seems be sudden and sure death. Anger, sadness, self-pity and being scared are definitely some of the feelings in the beginning. But those thoughts and emotions are joined by others and it all begins to weigh heavy on your shoulders.

Just as you begin to feel a little better about some part of your life, something else is tossed on top of all of the other baggage that you are carrying. Each new day of doctors, decisions and diagnoses seem to go by faster and faster. It almost comes to the point that if you think: *If I receive one more piece of information, I will fall down and never be able to get back up. This burden is too heavy.*

It's almost as if you are hiking and the farther up you get, the closer you get to your destination, more weight is put onto your back. You struggle to keep going since you think the biggest part of your journey is completed, until you top the hill to see that the destination is still too far away to see. I don't know how you would feel, but that's how I felt during the period of time from diagnosis to decision making. It never seemed to end.

Now, as I am able to sit back and reflect on that time of my life, I can see two things: First, that period of life seemed to go by so fast and secondly, it went by extremely slow. It seems ridiculous to say, "That time of my life seemed to go by so fast and so slow," but it did. I never felt like I had enough time, yet it felt like forever all at once.

What I mean is that the doctors visits and pondering over all the information about your condition never seems to stop. You carry this with you everywhere, everyday, trying to dissect all the information. It seems like it will never end. Yet, you have to make life altering decisions and appointments immediately! The next appointment or surgery are all too close and you feel like you don't have time enough to breathe, because of all of the decisions that have to be made, RIGHT NOW!

The aggravation and uneasiness don't seem to go away. Stress seems to continually build with each new step of the way. Because of that, time seems to speed by so fast that you don't feel you have time to sit back and just take a breath. On the other hand, even with all of the appointments and decisions that need immediate attention it never seems to end. Because you desire for it all to hurry up and come to an end, time seems to drag by.

Do you remember how excited you would get around Christmastime as a child? How each new day was getting you closer to opening your gifts? As exciting as that time was do you also remember how long it felt to get to Christmas day? I do. Even though each new day brought me one day closer to the end of waiting and ripping into those presents, it seemed like the 25th would never come. I was so excited to be done with my cancer treatments, and that part of my life, but the end date always seemed so far away. It felt almost unattainable and because of that, time seemed to drag by so slowly, it felt as if I would never see the end.

You may be wondering how I felt so much turmoil but never really feared death. As I mentioned before the only reason I wasn't concerned about dying was because of my faith. I understand that faith can consist of many components, different beliefs and can cover many different religions and ideologies, but the purpose of me writing about my cancer experience is to show what I felt and how I was able to deal with the news that I had cancer. I can only speak on what I believe and what helped me through my situation, so in order to understand where I am coming from, throughout this chapter and throughout the rest of this book, you must know that I am a Christian. I believe that Jesus Christ is God's Son, sent down to earth to take away my (and everyone who accepts Him) sins, so that I can have a relationship with my Creator.

Having shared that, some of you may not want to continue, but I urge you to keep reading if only for the simple fact that, in order to truly understand someone or how they have coped with something, you must first know the whole story. My whole story is just this, I truly believed and still do that no matter what happened – life or death – God had His hand on me and my life; and that His will would be done, no matter the outcome.

It is relatively easy to say this now, looking back over these events. As we all know, it is much more difficult to say this when you're right in the middle of upheaval. The main factor of being constantly able to handle myself in the mist of my cancer experience was to continue to look to God and to embrace His purpose for my life. My stability came from the way that I viewed my circumstances in relation to Him.

When faced with something seemingly as big as cancer it was helpful for me to look at something, or should I say someone, bigger. It helped me to put things back in perspective. Cancer was a big thing in my life, but my God was and is bigger! Not only is He bigger, He is Huge! He is wonderful! And, He cares for me!

Isaiah 40:12 always reminds me how big God really is:

> *"Who else has held the oceans in his hand? Who has measured off the heavens with his fingers? Who else knows the weight of the earth or has weighed out the mountains and the hills*?" (NLT)

Wow! That scripture always blows me away. The NIV translation reads:

> *"Who has measured the waters in the hollow of his hand, or with the breadth of his hand marked off the heavens..."*

In case you don't know what the breadth of your hand is, take your thumb and index finger and spread them apart from one another. That space between the two is the breadth. Can you see it now? That's really not a large area on our hand, but on the hand of God – He can hold the heavens in that space! He is huge! Compared to His hugeness, it may seem that we are so small. We may even feel insignificant in His eyes, yet He cares for us. That amazes me!

Another scripture that constantly blows me away is Matthew 10:30:

"And even the very hairs on your head are all numbered."

What? You mean to tell me that God knows how many hairs I have on my head? I know that some of us have more than others, but I can't even count the hairs on the top of my father's balding head! Yet God somehow knows! It amazes me that God is so big and I am so small and seemingly insignificant in comparison, yet He loves me anyway.

The greatness of God and His love for me is part of the reason that I wasn't fearful of dying. The other part may be a little harder to understand unless you're already on board with Jesus, so to speak. The other part is the assurance of my salvation.

To put it simply, while trying not to speak in Christianese, I know that when I die I'm going to be with God in heaven. For me, just to know that if I were to die I would be in a better place and feel no pain or have no more problems was wonderful. Understanding that not all people feel the same way about death and their resting place afterword, it is hard expressing my assurance that even if the worst would happen (death) that the best would be to come (heaven). For me, knowing that God loves me and that even if death did come as a result of my cancer, there is eternal life in heaven awaiting me. This is by far the main reason death did not and does not scare me.

Death has two commonalities no matter what you believe: First, it will happen. Second, no one knows when it will happen. Knowing this, I wonder why cancer seems to scare us? Is it death? While death is most associated with cancer, at the time of diagnoses, we don't know if that will even happen. The likelihood that I am going to die because of my cancer is just as probable as me getting in a car accident, just like the man I mentioned earlier. We just don't know when death will come and knock on our door. No one does or no one ever will.

Death will happen, but how it will happen is not for us to decide. When someone is diagnosed with cancer, yes, death will be a thought, but we must not let it dictate our lives or the lives of our family and friends. Death is certain, but cancer does not have to be the reason we die. As days go by, researchers and doctors are constantly finding new ways to treat and prevent cancer.

One day maybe there will even be a cure for it, but until that day comes we must not let ourselves get discouraged about our condition. We must over come and know that cancer is not necessarily a death sentence. I am a living example of just that.

Yes, there are always chances that I could get it again, but I cannot let that define me. Cancer can take away many things, but there are some things that it can't touch. Cancer can't take away your relationship with Jesus. Cancer can't take away your hope. Cancer can't take away your fight.

Even with modern medicine and treatments being more successful than ever before, there is another Hope. That hope is not found in researchers, doctors, or treatments; that hope is found in Jesus Christ. It is through our relationship with Him that we have hope, and through that hope we can keep fighting the good fight!

CHAPTER 5

Why Me?

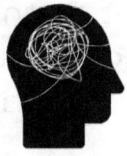

Things in life just happen. Sometimes we expect them and sometimes we don't. It's a part of life—although there are some things I wish would never happen. I can't understand why we get so upset at the things that we can't avoid, but we do. No one ever plans on getting a flat tire or stubbing his or her toe on the way to the bathroom in the middle of the night, but as soon as it happens what do we do? We get mad! There was no way to know that you would run over a nail or that the dresser would jump out in front of you in the dark of the night.

Do we really ever expect something bad to happen? I mean sure, we may plan on some things not going according to plan. We get insurance policies just in case, but none of us ever truly believe that disaster will happen. I guess it's just our human nature to never really expect bad things to happen, to us.

You may be just like me. When it's time to go somewhere, I get into my car, put on my seat belt and crank it up — I don't even give it a second thought. Am I right? Unless you've had car problems, like I have had before. Then each time you get in you say a little prayer that it will start as you turn key, but other than that, we just mindlessly get in and expect everything to work as it should. It's not something that we give much thought. So the day that the car doesn't start, it messes everything up. It's just human nature to expect the best, so when the unexpected comes along it messes up everything!

Every time I turn on the news something bad is happening. It's funny to me how it only seems like there are really two main things that most people are interested in when turning on the news: the weather and the traffic. And honestly, those aren't good half of the time either. The thing about watching the news is that even though we see all of the disaster and hardship that people are faced with, we really don't care.

Sure, we all feel a little sorry when the old woman falls down the steps trying to save Fluffy from her neighbor's dog, but almost as soon as the story is over we forget about grandma and go on with our lives. It's sad to realize how self-centered we really are, because if something doesn't directly affect us or someone that we truly care about…well…we probably could care less. Honestly, if I had never had cancer myself, I probably never would have cared about how people who are suffering with cancer feel either.

Thinking about that — how we could really care less about something or someone unless it directly affects us — seems selfish, but I know it is true. People come up and ask me to pray for them or to pray about something that's close to their heart because they know I am a Christian and believe in the power of prayer. So, when I'm asked, I pray for them… most of the time, but I'll be honest. Sometimes I forget. But, you know what I never forget to pray about when asked? The things that I have dealt with or struggled with, because at that point it becomes personal. I don't have to be reminded to pray for that person or their needs, because it hits home with me. I don't want them to struggle or feel the same anxiety, pain, or suffering I have felt in my life.

For instance, my parents got divorced when I was in my 8th/9th grade years, so when a young person tells me that their parents are having problems and may be getting divorced my heartbreaks for them. I remember back to when I was in a similar situation. I don't want that young person to have to face the heartache I felt. They don't have to ask me twice to pray for them, because I understand and relate to their pain.

On the other hand when 7th grade Susie comes to me and asks for prayer that her and her boyfriend 8th grade Eddie can work things out, it's a different story. It's just hard for me to diligently pray for a couple of middle school kids to be together forever. I mean lets be honest it's only going to last for a couple of weeks before they break up and are dating someone else anyway. It may sound bad, but I may or may not remember to pray for that situation like I would the first, because it doesn't hit home for me. I know that God cares for everyone in both of the scenarios, but when I can relate to a person it helps me better understand how to pray for them.

It has been that way ever since I was diagnosed with cancer too. The church we were a part of at the time of my cancer diagnoses had a prayer list (like every good Baptist church does). On that list was a whole section dedicated to cancer patients and I found my name in that section for a very long time. Before my name claimed its spot on that list, I can remember looking over that section of prayer requests and saying a quick, "God be with them" prayer, but no real feeling or emotions were attached to it. Was that wrong? Not really. I prayed and I meant it, but it was missing something – connection. It wasn't until I was dealing with my own cancer that I truly knew what it meant to have your name in that "special section" of the prayer list. At that point it was personal, I had a connection, I understood somewhat of what each of those people were going through. We may not have had the same type of cancer, the same treatment plan or the same recovery process, but we were connected.

I truly wish that I could have understood the emotions of being on the "special section" of the prayer list before I had cancer, but I didn't. You might be like I was at that time and just not know how someone feels because you have never been in a similar situation. Or you may be like I am now which is right the opposite, and you know exactly what it feels like to receive the news that you have cancer.

Regardless, we all have asked this next question at some point in our lives when things weren't going our way. And I can't think of a more appropriate time to ask it than when you have been told that you have cancer. You may be asking, *What is that question*? That question is... *Why me*?

I'm not sure I can really answer that question completely, or at least to your liking – nor mine for that matter. *Why do we get a flat tire? It should have been the guy who has been riding my bumper for the past five miles. I was the one driving safely; he is the one that deserves a flat tire not me.*

Why did I stub my toe on the dresser? Why couldn't it have been my wife? She probably deserves it more than me anyway (right guys?).

Who knows? But what I do know is that whatever is going on in those "why me?" moments, we certainly didn't ask for nor want bad things to happen. I, like many others before and after me, asked that same question when I found out that I had cancer.

Why me? I'm a good person. Sure I'm not perfect by any stretch of the imagination but I have never killed anyone or robbed a bank. I have never cheated on my wife. I'm a faithful churchgoer, I even teach Sunday school. What did I ever do to deserve this? Why me? Why couldn't it have been somebody who is in prison for murder or some other terrible crime? Why does it have to be me?

I would almost bet that just about everyone who has been faced with cancer has asked that question either audibly or internally. It's just human nature to wonder why something bad would happen to us.

Have you ever seen the movie *Forrest Gump?* I think it paints a great illustration of this "why me" mentality we have been talking about. Do you remember Lieutenant Dan? Lieutenant Dan was a true soldier. His whole family tree was full of soldiers, each who had died on the battlefield. His troop was in the middle of the jungle fighting the Vietnamese when a blast hit his legs. As the battle was still raging Forrest began carrying his wounded comrades to safety including Lieutenant Dan, who was unwillingly taken because he wanted to be left to die in battle like the rest of his family before him.

As the story continues, Lieutenant Dan had to get both of his legs amputated. He hated the fact that he had lost his legs and wasn't able to die on the battlefield. Basically, he was asking that same question – why me? To make a long story short, Lieutenant Dan eventually got over the fact that he did not die in battle and even learned how to use his prosthetic legs. At the end of the movie we see that he had gotten married and was now happy with the way that things had worked out. Like Lieutenant Dan, we can get upset and wonder why certain things happen to us, but the reality is that we may never know. That's why we must not let ourselves get upset and depressed because of a diagnosis. We have absolutely no control over getting or getting rid of our cancer. That is only decided by a higher power than you or me—our Almighty Creator.

Why me? Could it be because God has a special purpose for you and He is using this to help fulfill that purpose? Maybe it's something totally different, that's not for us to know, but maybe for us to figure out? I realize that I just gave a really lame answer for someone who has just received devastating news, but it is not a one size fits all answer. Just like we don't know why our car battery suddenly stops working even though it worked fine the day before, some things just can't be answered. Sure we can guess and sometimes we even will figure it out. Unfortunately with something like cancer it may not always be as simple as realizing you left your dome light on overnight.

Not everyone will have cancer for some special purpose. Can God use your cancer for good? Absolutely! But, lets be honest with ourselves. If I eat pizza and snack cakes everyday, and I get upset that I'm overweight and out of shape and then ask "why me?" I think I already have a pretty good answer. I want to be sensitive to the subject at hand, but sometimes we can help bring certain things onto ourselves. Since our topic is cancer, for instance, if I have been smoking for 30 years and then find out I have lung cancer – I might have a clue as to why.

Even still, it's okay to ask the question. Many people have done many things over the years that should have caused bad things to happen, but somehow they seem to walk away with no consequence. Yet others, feel that they didn't do anything to deserve their condition. No matter what, please understand that asking "why me" is perfectly okay, but what if we could ask a better question?

What if we were able to turn that "why me" or "why did this happen to me" into "how can God use me through my situation?" It's amazing how a slight change in our thinking can make a huge difference in our acceptance of something so bad.

During the time that I had cancer, Lance Armstrong was a name that resounded within the cancer community. He was a professional cyclist who was known for winning the Tour de France seven consecutive times (1999-2005) – the most in the event's history – all after recovering from testicular cancer. As you can imagine, I thought his story was great, especially being able to relate to the testicular cancer part. Lance shared that he had a very hard struggle in his battle with cancer, but he was able to overcome all odds and is now a living testimony of cancer survivorship. Because of his story and the national spotlight from cycling, Lance Armstrong was able to use his fame to really put cancer on the public's radar. I would be willing to bet that when he was going through his battle with cancer, Lance probably asked himself "why me" just like the rest of us. Even though he had a rough battle to overcome, he was able to utilize his platform (that God had given him) to help spread the word and champion the cause for cancer research.

Throughout the years, many people have been helped by research funded by his organization because rather than getting stuck in the "why me" stage, he was able to use his situation for something greater. If your familiar with the Lance Armstrong story you know that later he was stripped of his Tour de France titles and his reputation took a major hit after being involved in a doping scandal. Even still, he has had a huge impact on the cancer community simply by not allowing the "why me" mentality take ownership of his thoughts and life.

What I really think is important for us to remember is not to get stuck in a self-loathing, self absorbed, defeatist attitude because of our situation. It is so easy to let our concerns, our worries and stress take ownership. Those mindsets can cloud our vision, blocking out the good things that we actually have in our lives. I understand that it's so much easier said than done, especially when you are in the middle of something as life changing as cancer, but we need to try to look at the good, the positive things in our lives.

When we can see the good, even in the mist of bad times,

we can have hope. Hope, even in the confusion and chaos, can help us quiet the "why me?". I'm not saying it will magically go away, but it is so much harder to ask that question and feel sorry for yourself when you can see the positive all around you. Hope says that this too will pass and become a memory. Hope shows us that there will be some good in all of the confusion. Hope tells us that in the chaos we can have clarity.

Having a flat tire, stubbing your toe in the middle of the night or receiving the news that you have cancer can't even be compared to each other, yet we still seem to have the same "why me" mentality in each situation. I wish I could answer that question for you, but I can't even answer it for myself. Sometimes the question may not even have an answer and that's all right, because even in the unknown – I know the One who knows! I have hope, that even though I may not understand why, He does. My hope is in the Creator and even though I don't know why something is happening to me, He does. Because of that, I can have confidence that in His timing I will understand why it happened to me. As we close this chapter I want to leave you with some words of encouragement from Isaiah that can be applied into our lives today. I encourage you to personalize this verse because in doing so can really speak to your heart.

Isaiah 61:3 (NLT):

"To all who mourn in Israel [to Josh who is mourning], he will give a crown of beauty for ashes, a joyous blessing instead of mourning, festive praise instead of despair. In their [my] righteousness, they [I] will be like [a] great oaks that the LORD has planted for his own glory."

I HAVE CANCER?

CHAPTER 6

What Did I Do to Deserve This?

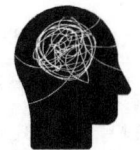

What did I do to deserve this? This question really goes hand in hand with our last question, "why me", but is something that I asked myself often during and after my diagnosis and treatment. I believe that this one single question resounds with so many people in the every day hardships of life as well. To be quite honest I don't know the answer to this question either.

Could it have been prevented? How can I keep this from happening again? What do I do now? Those are the types questions that pop into our heads in those moments where we feel we have no control. There is no sure answer to any of these questions, but in my personal experience, no matter what the answer, we must go on living. If we continue dwelling on what happened, we will never be able to let go of the problem.

I understand that this sounds so simple but in reality, it isn't. When I'm faced with a problem or a traumatic experience in my life, I am constantly reminded that it is always easier to talk the talk than to actually walk the walk. So many times as we talk to our friends and family we can give great advice, but if we really think about it, the advice that we give is always easier to talk about than it is to actually apply to our lives.

With that thought, I want you to know that what I'm trying to say, not only dealing with this particular question of "What did I do to deserve this?" but throughout the entirety of this book, is that *I know it's tough.* I know what I am trying to convey sounds so easy, but actually applying the correct attitude in order to "just go on with our lives" while dealing with problems and issues is really tough, especially when you are dealing with cancer.

So, what did we do to deserve cancer? I don't know. And you don't know either. Honestly, we may not have done anything to deserve it, but here we are. There are so many other questions in life that I wonder about and will never know the answer, but what I do know that there is a God who knows all the answers.

Bad things happen to good people. That's just life. I don't think that I had ever done anything bad enough to deserve cancer. I'm a good person. I never killed anyone, robbed a bank, cheated on my wife, so why did I get cancer? There are so many other people that are probably worse than me, but I'm the one who was diagnosed with cancer. I didn't deserve it, right? But, on the other hand do children deserve to starve to death or be beaten and raped by their parents or family members? Justice, in our minds, can appear... simple, almost cut and dry. For instance, if someone kills someone else, they deserve something bad to happen to him or her, right?

You may be thinking I'm a little crazy by now, but I hope you understand my point. Life isn't simple, but we have to keep moving forward. I know that doesn't necessarily sound great nor is that statement awe inspiring, but it is the truth. We may not like it, we may have done nothing to deserve it, but somehow we are facing something that we feel never should have happened to us. Now, before you completely write me off and stop reading let me point you to the story of a man named Job.

Job is a book in the Bible, and some believe Job to actually be the first book of the Bible written, even before Genesis. Job basically takes the reader on a journey through a portion of this man's life-changing experience, where he lost everything, including his family. Job was an extremely wealthy man, but was also labeled in the Bible as a blameless man of complete integrity. Job was a great guy who loved God, and his family, which consisted of his wife and ten children. As the story continues God pointed Job out to Satan and complemented him on his righteousness, but when Satan heard this, he immediately suggested to God that Job was only righteous because he was so blessed. God allowed Satan to take away Job's wealth, and even allowed his children to die; yet Job was still faithful. Job was tested again with a skin disease and even after some bad advice from friends, including his wife who told him he should just curse God and die, Job was still faithful. It was because of his faithfulness and devotion to God that eventually, after an unknown amount of time God blessed Job again with even more money, stuff and 10 more children.

You may be scratching your head by now wondering what in the world does that have to do with cancer or the question, "What did I do to deserve this?" I don't know Job personally nor do I know anything else about him except what I have read in the Biblical account with his namesake, but I'm pretty sure he probably asked a lot of the same questions that we have too. He may have even had more of a reason to ask them than we do. Who knows?

What I do know is that Job never expected that in such a short time he would lose his money, his possessions, and his children. Who would? The thing I love about Job is that even after such a traumatic loss like he experienced, he still praised God. I can't completely understand how he could have everything that any of us could want, lose it all, and still praise God.

I mean, when I get home from the drive-thru, open the bag and notice that my order is wrong, I get mad. At that moment I start to think, and sometimes even say out loud, "How hard is it to get the order correct?" They have computers to tell them what to fix, how many, what size, and even how much change to give me back when I pay. How in the world can something as simple as a hamburger get messed up? It's funny how something so simple can get us upset and at that moment we forget about everything else. Because our hamburger isn't the way we like determines that we have a bad day. How crazy is that?

Job, even after a huge life-changing event – not that he got pickles and mustard when he asked for ketchup and onions – but after losing everything, even his children, Job still praised God.

I realize that we don't have the luxury of seeing all of the emotion involved in Job's story or even how long it took for Job to be at the point where he could praise God, but I believe that he praised God in the mist of his troubles. I say that because even after losing all he had in life God allowed Satan to give Job a second test, a skin disease, because Job remained faithful throughout his loss.

The other thing about Job that I really admire is that even after the second test, the skin disease, he was still faithful. Now Job wasn't perfect by any means. He did do his fair share of complaining and even questioned God, yet that's why I really like him. Yes, we know him for his faithfulness and obedience to God, but he still is someone like me. He questioned, he wondered, he talked to friends about his problems, but after all was said and done, Job realized that he could not control any of the things that happened to him and went on with life.

I wish that all of our stories could end as well as Job's does and that we could get back everything and even more after our problem occurs, but I know that may not always be the case. In some instances once we think things are getting better, they get worse. Again, I don't have all the answers,

I HAVE CANCER?

I don't even have the answers to my own problems, but I know that we must keep going.

There is a phrase that I hear occasionally that makes sense but at the same time, it doesn't make sense. "When life throws you lemons, make lemonade." I'm sure that most of you have heard this phrase before in some way or another. Anyway, I understand where people are going with the statement and it does make sense, but you need a little more than lemons to make lemonade. In order to make lemonade you need lemons, sugar, water, and maybe even a pinch of lemon juice. Not only that but you need a pitcher for the juice, a knife, measuring cup, mixing spoon, cutting board, strainer and, well, you get the point. We need more than just lemons in order to make lemonade.

Maybe this isn't the best illustration I could have used, but in the way that it takes more than just lemons for a nice glass of lemonade sometimes God uses different things in our lives for his ultimate purpose. He may hand you the sugar before you get the water, and it may take a long time before he hands you the lemons. So we must be patient and realize that something like cancer doesn't have to be the end of our lives, it may just be the beginning of something we never could have imagined. You may have already been handed the cancer, but the people that you are going to comfort later may have not entered your life just yet. I may not know why we have things happen in our life – good or bad – but I know that God can use anything for His plan and purpose, and if your willing, He can even use you.

Job probably loved his life after all of the heartache was gone and he had more property, cattle, and money than he had before. He even had more children to "replace" the ones he had before (if I can even say that, since you can't ever replace a child). Life was good again for Job, but do I think he would have chosen this for his life? Or for his path to have gone the way it did? No, I don't.

If I knew that I was going to be diagnosed with cancer years before I would have been petrified. I would have tried to find a way out, or tried to make it where I could have avoided the whole situation all together. Thank God in all of His sovereignty and wisdom that we don't know what is going to happen next in our lives. If we did I wonder how many of us would be running around scared out of our minds trying to change the future? I know I probably would.

Yet because we don't know what each new day holds we have to learn how to deal with the problems that we will eventually face. Again, I know it sounds so easy, so why is it so hard? And again, I don't know, but I can tell you how I have learned to deal with things that I feel that I don't deserve. Believe me when I say that in no uncertain terms do I possess a secret formula to deal with problems, especially not cancer. But through all of my shortcomings I feel that I may be able to at least help comfort someone who has been in a similar situation. Just because you are in a bad time in your life doesn't mean it won't get better. Soon enough you may be able to look back at this moment in your life and realize that you got through it.

I know it's hard to have this mindset when we are going through hard times. To realize that these times won't last forever and that one day we will be able to look back at them. Quite honestly, even if we can embrace this line of thinking – it's hard to really apply those thoughts in our present pain.

I can only imagine that Job was in that limbo-land of thoughts as well. Just like us, he was getting all kinds of advice and words thrown at him through his friends and even his wife, some of those being good solid words of advice, while the others...not so much. Job seemed to understand that he needed to filter the good, solid advice from the bad. Even though just like Job our friends and family mean well, we need to make sure that we are filtering out the bad advice and more importantly that we sit, wait and hear what God is speaking to us.

In Job's case we see in chapters 38-41, that God does speak and when he speaks, Job knows it. When God steps into the picture to speak to Job he does it through a whirlwind. In His speech, The Lord asks Job several questions revealing His greatness. These questions help Job begin to understand how much he really doesn't know. God is showing His wisdom through everything that happens in life. It was through this time of listening to God that Job realized that even though he may not have done anything to deserve the things that happened to him, he may not have handled the circumstance as good as he thought. Job then repented and told God that he spoke out of ignorance.

I have said that it's all right to get angry and to tell God exactly how you are feeling and that is true. God is big enough to handle little me being angry and upset with my circumstances and even with Him. He is also big enough to take my yelling and crying at Him too, but just because He is big enough to take it, doesn't mean it was done appropriately.

Seeing Job's response to The Lord's criticism of how he was handling his present trials makes me understand that even though God allows us to be upset and vent our frustrations to Him, doesn't mean that I have done so appropriately. Many times in my life I have handled my aggregation of my present problems inappropriately, and spoken out of ignorance – just like Job. In these times I too need to repent just like Job did. Maybe you need to do that too?

When I feel that I haven't done anything to deserve the problems I am facing I get mad. I get angry. I yell. I don't handle things appropriately. I'm sure that I am not alone in my feelings either, you probably have done the same thing and that's okay. In 1 John we see that "God is faithful and just to forgive us" and I am thankful for that.

Even though we may not have done anything to deserve the hand we have been dealt and even though it is all right to be upset and question your circumstance, we need to be cautious in our actions. If we are not careful we can become so overwhelmed in our present circumstances that we can dig ourselves into a deeper hole of sorrow, worry and depression. When that happens, it is a lot harder and takes more time to pull ourselves out of the pit. Let's not let our past or our present dictate and determine our future.

Just like Job we can have a time of uncertainty, a time of questioning, a time of aggregation and anger, but lets be aware that even in those exaggerated feelings and emotions, we need to calm them, focus on what we can control and let God handle what we can't. He not only can, but He wants to. The question is whether or not we allow Him to handle it.

So, the question I have for you is this: What are you doing? Are you trying to handle everything on your own or are you giving it to Him? Too many times I have tried to handle the problems I faced by myself and too many times I realize that I can't do it on my own.

I understand that you may have family and friends in your corner and that's great, you need that! But sometimes, even when those we love are walking with us during our bad times, it doesn't seem to be enough. You still can feel alone and helpless, not knowing what to do, or where to turn next and it is because of that, I'm so thankful that God is with me too. There is something so comforting in that, even when we feel like we don't know what is going on in our lives.

Even when we don't know what we did to deserve the spot that we find ourselves in, God is there. Even when we can't see the future, the One who holds the future in His hands is with us, and if we allow Him – will lead us, and guide us through every circumstance we have in our lives.

I honestly do not know what I would have done or whom I would have turned to during the time of my life dealing with cancer without the Lord. Just knowing that even though I didn't know what the future held, He did – was life changing. It was Him who breathed new life in me and my circumstance even when I had no idea what to do. It was Him who gave me peace in unknowing times. It was Him who comforted me when I couldn't find comfort in the answers I was given. It was Him who was beside me when I felt all alone as thoughts flooded my mind. It was Him who allowed me to come out of a time in my life that I felt I didn't deserve, stronger and with a greater sense of purpose than I had before. And it was because of Him allowing something to happen to me that I would have never wanted or asked for, that my faith in Him has grown.

In all of that, I can now look back at that time in my life, where it felt as if my life was falling apart, as something I am grateful to have happened to me. Not that I would ever want to go back and experience it again, but I am thankful that I was able to grow from it as a man and in my relationship with God.

It may seem so far fetched for you to believe that you can one day look back at your cancer as a blessing, but I have learned that the farther away we get from the things we have faced in our past, the more we can appreciate what we learned from it. I hope that you too can look back at your experience with cancer, and see that even though you may not have deserved it, you grew from it and perhaps, you are even better for it.

CHAPTER 7

What about Jamie?

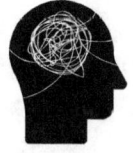

At some point in everyone's life we think about death – cancer or not – and it is in those times that we reflect on what we have done in our lives and what it will be like for others when we are gone. I don't know at what point that happens for everyone, but for me it was after I found out that I had cancer. I was still young and felt like I had a whole lifetime ahead of me, until I didn't. It's amazing how quickly our mindsets can change when certain things happen. I'm not saying that we never think about death. Maybe we don't think about it as much when we are younger, but there seems to be a natural progression, as we get older to think about it more. Even still it isn't necessarily a pleasant thought, regardless of age, but for whatever reason, whenever we begin to think about us not being on this earth, it definitely brings forth a lot of different thoughts and emotions.

For me, I knew that at some point I would eventually die, *eventually* being the key word. I was young, I was newly married and I had big plans for what my future was going to hold. Death wasn't even on my radar; I just wanted to have fun, enjoy my wife, my family and my friends. Nothing else really seemed to matter, especially not death. It was during this exciting season that I was told that I had cancer and all of those plans came to a screeching halt. I was thrust into thinking about something I thought was so far off, something I shouldn't have to think about for fifty more years! Even still, here I was.

All of my life, up until the time that I was married, I only had to think about myself. Being an only child I never had a bond with siblings like so many others do. My relationship with my parents was good but they didn't rely on me for anything, so I only had to worry about myself. Let's be honest for a second though, we all are extremely selfish and really only think about ourselves most of the time. But for the first time in my life I started to worry about someone other than myself. I was a newlywed. When I learned that I had cancer, I began to worry about my wife. *What about Jamie? What's she going to do? How will she handle her husband dying? She's going to be a widow!*

Among all the thoughts that I was contemplating, this one may have been the hardest to consider. Like I said, we were just starting out in our marriage journey. Now it felt like I was going to be checking out early. "Til death do us part" felt like it was closer than either of us would have expected. Even as much as I felt that everything was going to work out and I was going to be okay, this was weighing heavily on my shoulders.

In some weird way, I felt like I was betraying her somehow, by marrying her just to leave her alone so soon. I finally was worrying about someone other than myself, feelings that I had never really felt before. And as cheesy as it may sound, I felt like I was her protector and that I would not be able to protect her anymore if I didn't make it. Looking back now with 15 years of marriage under my belt, she would have been just fine.

She didn't need me to protect or provide for her, she was doing just fine before I ever entered the picture, and maybe even more so now, but when you love someone it doesn't matter if they need you or not, you want to protect them, provide for them, care for them and support them no matter what. That is how I felt. I didn't want to leave my wife as a widow in her mid-20's and honestly, didn't want to think about her moving on and finding someone who wasn't me.

It's funny how priorities and perspectives change throughout the different stages of your life. If I would have been diagnosed before I was married, I'm sure that I would have asked all of the same questions that we have already discussed, but they may not have carried the same weight. I wouldn't have wanted to die, but marriage changed the way I lived my life.

If you aren't married, you probably won't truly grasp what I'm trying to convey here, but with each new stage, new worries come with it. This worry – worrying if I would be here for my wife – was one that I was experiencing for the first time and I didn't like it at all.

I don't consider myself a very jealous husband probably because my wife has never given me any reason to be. Even still, the thought that I would not be in Jamie's life and that she may find someone else didn't sit well with me. Not that I wouldn't want her to be happy, but she is my wife and the thought that she would or could love someone else was actually painful to think about.

I also had this new, unspoken assignment – that it is my job to protect her. Even though I know that I can't keep bad things from happening to her, or keep hurt and disappointment from her heart, it is my desire to try. I'm not some huge muscle bound guy who knows mixed martial arts; but I want to protect her if someone were to try to physically harm her. And even so more when it comes to protecting her heart. I understand that I am unable to protect her from hurt feelings, but I sure want to. It's weird. I never planned on feeling that way, but I do. I love her and because of that I want to protect her however I am able. So the thought that I may not be there to protect her was very hard to think about.

Now that I am older and we have had our son, I know that those feelings would be even greater. I have heard so many stories and read so many different statistics about the effects on children who are being raised without both parents in their lives, especially without their fathers. I understand how important it is for children to have both parents involved in their lives. Knowing this, I assure you that I would have felt that same desire to protect Jonathan, maybe even more so.

Losing a parent, especially in the younger years of the child's life can be very hard for the children to deal with. Because of this, I can't imagine dealing with the burden of those thoughts as well. I'm sorry if you have ever had to wrestle with the thoughts and emotions of leaving your child parent-less. I can't fathom having to deal with that. Thankfully I didn't have to deal with that during my time with cancer.

Right now someone I know has been diagnosed with terminal cancer and their doctors have actually put a timeline on their life. Thankfully, so far they have beaten the given timeline, but now they feel like they are living on borrowed time. I'm so grateful that when I received the news of my cancer that I didn't have a timeline attached to it, but unfortunately for many that is not the case. I don't know how I would have taken that news but I'm pretty confident that I wouldn't have taken it well. If that is you or someone that is close to you, please know that I mourn for you. My hope is that you can enjoy the time you have or the time you can spend with them here on earth before eternity.

I pray that this is not taken the wrong way, because I would not want that to happen, but just now I had a thought – even though you may have a timeline on your life, which is terrible news, there might be something good that can come from this news. Even others can benefit from reading this thought. Knowing that the end of life is coming would inevitably shift our life perspective. We need to make sure that we are living our lives to the fullest, enjoying each day as it comes because we never know when we will breathe our last breath on this earth. We need to make sure that our relationships are taken care of and that we have not allowed bitterness and strife take ownership of our lives. We need to resolve our issues and strive to live in peace with one another – our family, friends and neighbors.

My last thought is that we need to make sure that the people we love know that we love them. None of us are promised tomorrow, cancer or not, so let's start living our lives in a way that we want to be remembered.

I understand that everything that we have been talking about throughout our time together can be very sensitive in nature, but especially our current topic. Because of that before we go any further into our discussion, I would like to take a moment and pray for you:

> *Father, I come to you right now and ask for you to give my friends peace in their lives. I don't know what they are going through in this moment of time, but you do. You are the master architect behind each and every life and nothing is a surprise to you. You know where they are in their lives right now, you know and understand the hurt, pain, anguish and heartache that they may be feeling and I ask that you comfort them in this time.*

> *They have probably asked many of the same questions and have felt the same discouragement that I have, and I ask you to be with them just like you were with me. I know that I'm not alone in my feelings of fear; that the people that I feel that I need to protect may end up alone and that I may not be there with them. It is a very lonely place, and I ask that you fill that hole in their lives with your Spirit.*

Help us to live our lives in a way that is pleasing to you. Help us to remember that we are not promised tomorrow and have never been promised tomorrow and that because of that we should strive to live our lives in peace with everyone.

Lastly, Father, I want to ask that those who are reading this who do not know you as their personal Lord and Savior will be open to hearing from you in this moment. Thank you for loving us and for always being beside us even when we don't deserve it. I ask these things in the mighty name of Jesus, Amen.

Thank you for allowing me to pray for you.

Talking about the fear of leaving my wife may seem like a weird topic to discuss when talking about the fears, questions and emotions associated with cancer. However, I truly believe that I'm not the only one who has felt this way towards my wife – or anyone else that we love and feel a sense of commitment towards.

I like that word – commitment. Maybe this is a better way to express what you may be feeling. I did feel and continue to feel that I am a protector to my wife and now my son, but there is also a sense of commitment as well.

We may not necessarily think about the husband/wife, parent/child relationship in terms of being a commitment specifically, but we should. When we speak those wedding vows or help bring a new life into the world, we are committing to see it through. It's a commitment of love, of faithfulness, to provide and to protect. I'm sure we can name many more, but when contemplating your death, these are real things we think about making the thought of leaving more real, hurtful and painful than many can imagine.

Many thoughts can float around in our minds when we have received bad news or are dealing with unforeseen circumstances. I want to point out three different questions that many of us think about when contemplating our death.

The first question that I want to address is one that we have already been talking about. I understand that we have already discussed this to a degree, and I won't focus too much more on it, but I do think it is an important question that the majority of people seem to have when contemplating their death.

What will they do when I'm not there? Like everything we have discussed so far, this is not a cut and dry nor a black and white answer. Each situation is different and each relationship, whether family or friend, is different too. Because of this we really don't know what the ones we love will do when we are gone, nor can we control it.

One thing I have witnessed is that when people lose someone close to them, they usually are able to continue living. Of course, there is a period of grief. Possibly even a time of confusion mixed with a bit of chaos because everything changes, but after this season they are able to go on living their life. Sure, things are different when a loved one is missing from their daily lives, but unfortunately death is a certainty in this life and God has designed us in a way to be able accept what has happened and continue living our lives.

I don't mean to be insensitive to the subject, but I understand that death isn't something new. And even though my death may be upsetting to a few people, I know that they will be able to cope and move on with their lives. Like I mentioned, God designed us to be resilient beings, able to handle whatever happens in this life. 1 Corinthians 10:13 (NLT) says,

"The temptations in your life are no different from what others experience. And God is faithful. He will not allow the temptation to be more than you can stand. When you are tempted, he will show you a way out so that you can endure."

This scripture has been and continues to be taken out of context by a lot and people say that God will not give you more than you can handle (referring to numerous things in life). But Paul is writing about temptations towards sin. Even though he is referring to sin and it's temptations in our lives, I believe that this principle applies to other parts of our lives. I believe that principle can apply to our current conversation as well.

When we deal with the death of someone close to us we walk thorough stages of grief, and I believe that in each of those different stages of grief we may be tempted to sin by not trusting in God's grand provision. But as we see from this verse in 1 Corinthians, God will not allow us more temptation than we can stand. Because of that, I know that we can overcome our feelings of grief, loneliness and abandonment – because God is with us, and He will not allow us to be tempted more than we can handle so that we can resist sinning.

Do we know what our loved ones will do when we aren't there? No, but we can be assured that they are not alone. God is with them and He will not abandon them. Yes, there will be pain from our loss, but just like so many others before us and so many after, they too will be able to continue with their lives all while having the memories of us in them.

That leads me to the next question that many of us have: *Will others remember me?* Short answer, "Yes."

For a slightly longer answer: When we are contemplating

our death and wondering if others will remember us, we can look back and remember the loved ones that we have lost who have not been forgotten.

Each day, you and I have many experiences to remember. Those memories include things we have done and the people that we have shared life with. Not every memory is one that makes us proud and we may not even consider all of them good. Still, there are other memories that we can look back on and enjoy, laugh about and cherish. There are some moments in our lives that seem terrible at the time, but when we look back at them, they become laughable, and we may even be glad that they happened. These memories allow us to reflect, to look back on the things that have shaped our lives and helped us to become the person we are today. So, just as we can remember different times and people in our lives, our loved ones will too. You will be remembered; it's *how* you are remembered that matters most, and that is up to you.

That leads us to our last question, which is – *What purpose did my life serve*? This is the question that really hits home with me, both when I was really contemplating my life during my season of cancer and probably even more so now. Everyone wants to leave some sort of legacy. At what degree and magnitude may differ, but everyone wants to be remembered for something. It could be that you want to be remembered as a good husband or wife, a wonderful father or mother, a successful businessperson, a fan of a particular team, a lover of nature, a respected employee or a ton of other things – the point being we all want to be remembered by something.

I guess what we need to figure out is what we want to be remembered for and make sure that we are living our lives in a way that will allow that to happen.

I'm not naive to the fact that on my deathbed I will have some regrets. Things that I wish that I could go back and fix or things that I should have never done, and in all likelihood you will too. I also understand that sometimes in life we may not get to do everything that we had planned or wanted to due to an array of circumstances. Finances, time, changing priorities and so many other obstacles can derail the plans and ambitions for our lives, but it doesn't mean that our lives were for not.

Rather, I want to remind you of something I said a bit earlier. All of the experiences in our lives, the good and the bad, have molded and formed who we are right now. We may not necessarily feel that each of those experiences were for the best, yet the people we love and care for still love and care for us. They are in our lives because we are worthy of their time, energy and love.

While we may have different dreams and desires in our lives that we were never able to fulfill, it's all right. Your life is still meaningful. You still have been a blessing to someone, and you will be remembered.

The only thing that we can control is our next step. So, I encourage you, if you still have breath in your lungs and a heartbeat in your chest, strive to fulfill what God has for your life. We will never find satisfaction in life until we submit to His plan and purpose. Through pursuing Him we will leave a legacy that will last long after we are gone.

CHAPTER 8

Again?

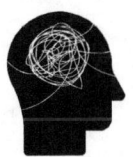

I am not sure at what point it comes, but eventually, your cancer story starts to fade away and you think less and less about it. It never really goes away. You have moments when you still think about it. You talk about it when the subject is brought up, but it becomes less important over time. I'm sure that everyone's timetable is different but at some point, just like anything else in your life, cancer doesn't consume it.

After a year of being cancer free you are officially considered in remission. After my surgery and chemo treatments, a couple of months of clear CT scans and good blood work, I was told by my Oncologist that I was officially cancer free and in remission. When you hear those words come from the mouth of your doctor, it feels as if a huge burden was lifted off your shoulders. That is exactly how I felt.

Even being officially in remission, I wasn't out of the woods just yet. I had to have CT scans every three months for the first year that I was cancer free, then it went to every six months, then to once a year and now I don't have to have them at all. Along with the CT scans came blood work, so every time I went to my Oncologist to get my results of my scan, I had blood work done as well. The scans were important, but even more important was the blood work. As you may remember, my blood work is where it was first discovered that I had cancer. With as many doctors' visits, blood draws and CT scans that I have had, you can probably imagine that it just became routine. I didn't think much about it after a while. It was just another appointment, visit or stick in the arm and they always came back fine – until one day it wasn't fine.

It was October 12, 2010, almost one year after I was in

remission that everything changed – again. Like I said, it was just another doctor's visit like the seemingly hundreds I'd had before, so there was no need to worry. Just go in, talk to the doc, get my good results, pay for the visit and get on with life. And that's usually just what I did.

At that time, my job included visiting a territory of grocery stores. That day, midway through my day I had an appointment with my Oncologist to review the results from my CT scan and have my blood drawn. I went to my appointment and as expected my CT scan came back great with nothing to worry about. After talking to my doctor, I went to the phlebotomy area to have my blood drawn and I then was off to call upon my stores.

Typically, the doctor's office would call me about two weeks later to let me know that the results of my labs came in and everything was fine. That's what I expected to happen that day too. Unfortunately, not too long after I hopped into my car and was heading down the interstate my phone rang, and it was my doctor's office calling. I thought it was strange but figured that I may have left something at the office or something may have gone wrong with my payment. Never did I ever expect the news that I was about to receive.

"Mr. Gladden, the results of your blood work came back and you have cancer."

"What!!?? Can you say that again please? Did I hear you correctly? You said I have cancer...again!!??"

I can't explain the flood of emotions that came over me, but that burden that had been lifted off my shoulders was back, and bigger than ever! I'm not sure what happened after I got off the phone. All I remember was driving down Interstate 20 going towards Atlanta, thinking, *I've got to go back to work.*

I HAVE CANCER?

I was in total shock and didn't know what to do. I wanted to go home, but I didn't want to go home. I wanted to continue with my workday to feel like everything was normal, but I didn't want to work. I called my wife and told her the news. I don't remember any of our conversation.

After that I called my parents to tell them the news. I remember my dad asking me where I was. I told him I was driving down the interstate towards a store that happened to be right down the road from his office and that I didn't know if I should go home or not. He asked me to meet him in the parking lot of the store and I did.

I vaguely remember being in a hazy state of mind as I pulled into the very back of the parking lot. I sat there, watching cars drive past on the main road in front of the store. At some point my dad pulled up and got into the passenger's seat of my car and we began to talk. The only part of our conversation I remember was me telling him, "Why did it have to be me? I already had to deal with this, so why do I have to do it all again? I'm a good person, why couldn't have been someone else?"

Funny how those same questions came up again, huh? It's crazy, but it's true. I was so confused, so aggravated, so mad that I had cancer again. I couldn't understand it. Why me? Again?

The only other thing that I remember from that day was that after my conversation with my dad I went home. It was so weird hearing those words again. I can't describe the sinking feeling in my stomach when I heard the news. It was so unexpected, not like hearing those words are ever really expected, but I thought that chapter of my life was over. Yet here it was back again for a second go around.

I know that not all cancer is the same and many people can

suffer with recurrences of their cancer, but for me this was a total shock. The type of cancer that I had wasn't supposed to come back. Not to be too graphic, but when you get testicular cancer, it can only be in one area and there are only two places it can go – the right side or the left side. I haven't heard of anyone who has experienced it in both testicles at the same time, not saying that it hasn't or won't happen, but that would be a rare occurrence.

One of the reasons I was in such shock at the news that I had cancer again was because with testicular cancer there was only a 1% chance that you would ever get it for a second time. Knowing that, I assumed that I was home free and would never get it again. Nope, not the case, I don't know if I've ever been in the 1% of anything in my life and probably never will be again, but here I am! I am the 1% of people who get testicular cancer two times in their lives! Lucky me....

Well after the news, I had to go back to the urologist because another surgery was going to be needed to take out my other testicle. If you remember, we didn't care too much for my last urologist, so my wife and I decided we were going to find someone else this time around and we did. My wife had made it her mission to find me another urologist that specialized in reproductive urology and she did. The doctor that she found was amazing. Not only did he specialize in reproductive urology, but he specifically specialized in testicular cancer.

The first visit my wife went along to meet the new doctor and listen to the surgery plan. We were both impressed by him. He was intrigued by my case and asked if he could share my information with his four colleagues who shared the practice with him. None of them had seen someone who had testicular cancer twice – yep, there's that 1%. I was more than glad to grant him permission because I thought the more doctors who were looking at my case the better. If someone overlooked something, hopefully someone else would catch it and I figured it couldn't hurt.

The only bad thing I could say about my new urologist was that his office wasn't too convenient. From where we lived it could take around an hour to an hour-and-a-half to get to his office and to the hospital that he worked out of. That being said, I am very grateful that I didn't let the time or distance scare me away from having him as my physician.

I mentioned earlier not to let anyone or anything influence your decision on finding the right physician for you. This is why I truly believe that: I could have gone back to my first urologist. He did perform a successful surgery, his office was very convenient, as was the hospital he worked from. However, his lack of bedside manners, lack of patient care, and lack of information sealed the deal for us. We determined to move on to another doctor for my second surgery.

My second urologist was the exact opposite in every way. He had fabulous bedside manners, he truly seemed to care about me as his patient and would give us all the information that he had. If we had questions about something he made sure that if he didn't have the answer at the time, he would get it for us. On top of that he was a better surgeon.

After my second surgery, which was the same surgery that I had the first time, except on the opposite side, I was off for my second time of chemo treatments. As you can imagine, they were just as bad as the first time, only this time I knew what to expect. We did the same exact treatment plan as before, with the same three chemotherapy drugs, Bleomycin, Cisplatin and Etoposine. I also had to take the same white blood cell booting shot of Leukine on the days I wasn't receiving my treatments, although this time my body decided that it didn't like the Leukine and I had an anaphylactic reaction to it.

I had just finished my chemo treatments and my wife and I went to visit my mother-in-law who was serving in the Army and was stationed in Washington, DC at the time. I was pretty much forbidden by my oncologist to be around large groups of people because my immune system was so weak. So I stayed at the house while my wife and her mom got to go spend time together. While we were visiting, I started feeling a little bad and the next thing I know my body was covered head to toe in hives. I went to an emergency clinic and was given some steroids to fight the reaction, but there were a couple of miserable days I had to deal with.

After I got back home, I went to see my oncologist. She kept a very close watch over me to make sure we didn't have any more issues or reactions to the medication I had to take.

When taking treatments like chemotherapy, you could have a myriad of reactions. Sometimes they are immediate while others take time to develop. After my second time dealing with cancer and the treatments I began to notice some differences. I had never had a reaction to any sort of medication before I had my incident with the Leukine injections. Even before I had my anaphylactic reaction, my stomach would get red, inflamed, sensitive to touch and very itchy at the injection site. I also have developed some food allergies. I was never allergic to anything – food or medication before chemo. Not only have I had allergic reactions to medicine and food since receiving chemotherapy treatments, but my taste for certain foods is different now as well.

I understand that I am getting older and with age your food likes and dislikes do change, but what I'm referring to happened almost immediately after my treatments began.

Suddenly, I could not stand sweets. Before, I couldn't get enough of them – candy bars, snack cakes, donuts, you name it I loved them. It's only now, some 10 years removed, that I am enjoying them again, but not nearly as much as before.

My hair is different too. After losing my hair during treatments, it came back curly. Now it has straightened back similarly to what it was before, but the color is a shade different – and I'm not including the newfound gray either. I've even got this random circular blonde spot in the back of my head that my wife points out now. So, I have experienced some internal and external changes in my body since receiving chemo, nothing too crazy or too bad, but definitely some things that I have to be cautious about when taking new medications or eating certain foods.

There were a few other changes in my medical care, so daily life changed a bit after my second time with cancer. As you can probably guess after chemo I had to start back on my CT scan and blood work schedule, but the first "new" was that I had to add another doctor to my "team" of medical professionals. Because of the type of chemotherapy and the dosages that I had to take both times, which was very bad for my lungs, my oncologist felt that it was important for me to see a pulmonologist in order to monitor my lungs.

I remember that visit, the day my oncologist was telling me about having to see a pulmonologist. She asked me if I smoked. I didn't and I told her so. She was glad because smoking would only hasten any issues that I may have with my lungs. After that, she looked at me very intently and asked if smoked "the marijuana". It seemed kind of funny and I assured her that I didn't. She continued looking at me intensely and said very sternly, "Good, because that would be like instant death."

To me that was such a funny moment because of the way she asked about it and I guess because I didn't smoke anything including "the marijuana" that made it even more comical to me.

I saw that pulmonologist for a couple of years. She was a very good doctor, very thorough and very nice. I would have to go in a few times a year and do breathing a test. I don't know if it was my lungs or just me, but that thing wasn't for the weak of lung, that's for sure. I was young and had pretty good lungs outside of the beating from the chemo, but it wasn't a fun little exercise. Luckily, after a couple years of monitoring, I was given the okay and haven't had to see a pulmonologist since.

The last thing that changed and is something that I still do daily is that I now must take testosterone. Being that I had testicular cancer two times, I can no longer produce my own testosterone. In case you don't know, men produce their testosterone from their testicles. Being that mine were both surgically removed means I must supplement my testosterone. It was my 2nd, and best, urologist that informed me that I would need to get my testosterone levels checked and be put on some sort of a supplemental medication to keep my body functioning as it should. He suggested that I find an Endocrinologist to check, prescribe and maintain a close look at my testosterone levels, which I continue to this day. Currently, I am down to only seeing my Endocrinologist every three to six months. The blood work they do includes checking my tumor markers and of course my testosterone levels.

I don't want to bore you with too much information that may not be relevant to your particular situation, but I think it could be beneficial to see what someone else has gone though. I also want to show you that even throughout that season of diagnosis, treatment and initial remission that things do eventually seem to slow down and become less life consuming and more of a distant memory.

As you can see, I am still dealing with the effects of my cancer, but I don't think much about it at this point. While I still have to get my blood work and take medication that I wouldn't have had to otherwise, it has just become a part of my daily life. .

And I know that even if cancer is currently flooding your thoughts and dictating your life, one day you too will be able to look back at this moment in your life as a memory and see that you have overcome it. For me to receive the news that I had cancer again for a second time, initially was a huge punch in the gut, but once I remembered that I had already gotten through it once, I knew that I could do it again. The thing that really helped was already knowing the process and treatment that I would be doing.

I understand that not everyone is as fortunate as I was having the same type of cancer and treatment. The unknown of a different type of cancer, one that you are unfamiliar with can be very unnerving. Yet I believe there is a sense of assurance in knowing that you have been in a similar circumstance and come out of it once before. I really believe that in this knowledge there can be peace. Whether it is accomplishing a similar task or, in this case, surviving another type of cancer there is hope that you will do it again.

It is always good to look back throughout our lives and see what we have accomplished or what God has helped us overcome. Those reflections of our past can give us hope for our future. If we did it once before, we can surely do it again and if God was with us before, He will surely be there again!

CHAPTER 9

Dealing With Disappointment

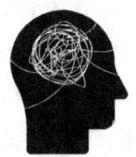

Disappointment may not be a feeling that one would initially associate with a cancer diagnosis, and honestly, I didn't either. It has taken some years and much reflecting on my experience to begin to really understand that I carried a sense of disappointment along with me for quite a while. I don't believe that I'm alone in that feeling.

I couldn't see it. In the initial shock and flood of emotions I didn't really realize or even understand that disappointment existed there too. I'm sure that I am not alone in this feeling, although it may manifest itself in some of the other emotions that we are experiencing at the time as well. Because of the flood of emotions, we may not always associate disappointment in our cancer story. However, I believe that understanding that the disappointment exists could be very beneficial as we are enduring our diagnosis and treatment. I also think that it is important for those supporting a person dealing with a cancer diagnosis to understand that among the many emotions that their loved one is experiencing they may also be dealing with disappointment. When we understand that disappointment may be present, we can better deal with or support someone in this stressful time in their lives.

I understand that disappointment may look different for each person, but for me the initial disappointment was the realization that I actually had cancer. I know that may be odd to hear, disappointed that I had cancer, but it is true. I was disappointed because it is something that was never on my radar when it happened. Strangely, it was as if I was almost upset with myself that "I allowed" this to happen to me. I understand that sounds weird too, since there wasn't anything, I could have done differently to have stopped or prevented getting testicular cancer. It wasn't like I was doing something that would have caused my cancer to manifest, it just happened. I guess that feeling that I had of "allowing myself" to have cancer came from the aggravation that I had it. I was trying to put the blame on something but I couldn't place it on anything. The real disappointment was that it had happened to me.

This led to another aspect of disappointment, which was the realization that I was going to have to deal with this the rest of my life. I felt that my whole life would be clouded by my cancer diagnosis and that cloud would loom heavy over my life for as long as I lived. Understandably so, because at the time, it was something that I thought about almost all day, every day. *What was the next step? What was the next plan of action? What did I need to take care of? How much was this going to cost? How long will this last?*

Looking back, it wasn't nearly as long as it felt, but when something like that is heavy on your heart and mind it doesn't ever seem like it will go away. Yes, I am still dealing with the fact that I have had cancer to this day. I still must see a doctor I wouldn't have otherwise, but in the whole scheme of life, the whole thing doesn't really seem that bad. I just wish I would have known that back then.

I was not only disappointed that I had cancer and I was going to have to deal with it the rest of my life, but I was also disappointed that my plans were going to have to change. It seems silly to think about, but no one likes to have their plans changed, especially unexpectedly (remember I'm the nerdy control freak). It's aggravating when you have plans to be somewhere or do something at a certain time on a particular day and you get a phone call that says that those plans are going to be delayed or even worse, they have been moved forward.

If you're anything like me when we are getting ready to

go out of town, I have a checklist of things to do in order to leave at the determined time. This means bags packed and loaded, set time to wake up, get ready and head out. Inevitably something happens to delay our departure and I get aggravated. As insignificant as that may be, imagine how cancer messed up my potential future plans. How it would have shaken me up. Even though it was out of my control, it was disappointing to me that life had to change immediately and potentially those changes would affect my future. Disappointing, especially since I didn't want this change in the first place!

The last real disappointment that I faced was that I may not have the option of having children. Even though my wife and I didn't want kids when we first got married, we liked keeping our options open. The first time I was diagnosed with cancer we were unsure if we would ever be able to conceive because of the possible lymph node removal surgery we discussed in an earlier chapter, along with the fact that I was going to be losing half of my baby producing organs. So, there was a real concern about that at the time.

After my second time having testicular cancer the option would be gone completely. I'm sure you can understand – when something is taken away from you – even if you will never need, want, or use it – it's disappointing. When you have choices and suddenly the option is no longer available, it can be a let down. And that is where I found myself, disappointed. I know it's easy to look back now and say, "There's nothing you could do about it. Don't worry about it." And honestly, I knew those things then too. It's just hard sometimes to motivate yourself to see that and even harder sometimes to believe the truth when you are so upset, worried, scared and disappointed in the situation that you find yourself in.

We need to be careful to not let disappointment creep into our lives as much as possible because disappointment can lead to fear. I'm not just talking about the fear of dying or the fear of what pain or side effects a treatment may cause. The type of fear that I am referring to here can make itself known in a few different ways.

The first way I believe it shows itself to us is in the fear that things that have happened in our past will happen again. I'm sure that it doesn't come as much of a shock to you if you haven't ever had cancer – and if you have, I bet you have thought the same way too – that there is a fear that you will get it again. I honestly don't know if there is a way not to be a little scared of that if you have had cancer. It seems to be a logical thought and I know that I had it after both times that I had cancer. I will say that after both of those times that the thought of getting cancer again did seem to go away pretty quick after the first couple of times my blood work came back clear. I'm not saying that I don't occasionally have the thought about having to experience cancer again, even today, but if and when I do have those thoughts, they fade away fast because I don't allow them to consume my mind anymore. It's natural to think that something that has happened to you will happen again, but we can't let those thoughts of something that may not ever come to fruition take precedence in our minds. Too many times we allow our present to be dictated and determined because we are fearful of what could or could not happen in our future.

Fear can also manifest itself through disappointment because we may not be able to accomplish something we thought should be done because cancer put our plans on hold. Or maybe it could be that we believe that we may never be able to accomplish what we put on hold, ever, because the opportunity may have been passed up for good.

I HAVE CANCER?

Those are both ways that we can be disappointed, when things don't go the way we planned or we feel that we may not have certain opportunities available to us again. That is true not only in the stresses of cancer, but in life altogether. When we feel that we have missed opportunities it can be disappointing, and that can easily be turned into fear that they will never happen again.

The thoughts of not being able to have children really helps this point come to life. My wife and I were fearful. We started to wonder if we may have missed the window for having children. Even though kids weren't on our radar at the time, the thought that we may not have the ability to have them was a pretty hard pill to swallow. I don't think that either of us verbalized those words to the other at first, but the conversations eventually took place about what our future may hold in that area.

During my first time with cancer we decided it was best if we "banked" my sperm in case I may not be able to bear children. I don't want to veer off topic too much here, but it's not like I haven't already told you any other embarrassing facets of my experience. Some of you may be wondering what I'm talking about "banking" my sperm. Just so you know what I'm talking about, we had to collect my sperm and send it off to a laboratory so they could cryogenically freeze it and store it for us. This was in case I became sterile after my surgery and treatments. If Jamie and I decided that we would like children of our own we could use my own specimen to fertilize Jamie's eggs. Seeing the process of what we had to do, I'm sure you can understand how we were disappointed in our situation – and even how that disappointment lead us to fear what might happen in the future.

If we are not careful, we can allow disappointment and

fear to take control of our lives, without even knowing it. Fear is a crazy thing; it can cause us to shut down and stop trying before we even start something. It can make us give up plans, dreams and ambitions because it causes us to believe the lies it puts into our heads about our situations and circumstances. I have known many people over the years, myself included, who gave up on dreams and desires because of fear. Fear of the unknown, fear of failure, fear of what others may think, do or say. Fear can crush our dreams and our God given purposes if we allow it. Fear can cripple us and do you know what fear leads us back to? That's right, it comes around full circle, right back to disappointment. Fear can cause us to give up on whatever our dreams, desires and purpose may be; and when we give up on those things, we become disappointed. Disappointed in our circumstances. Disappointed in the things that may never happen. Disappointed that we didn't accomplish what we wanted to. It's a crazy cycle that, if we are not careful, can be debilitating to our lives.

Disappointment not only leads to fear, but disappointment also can lead to discouragement. It's like a trifecta of terrible thoughts, feelings and emotions that are all trying to take control of your mind, and your life.

Isaiah 41:10 (NLT) says:

> *"Don't be afraid, for I am with you. Don't be discouraged, for I am your God. I will strengthen you and help you. I will hold you up with my victorious right hand."*

In this verse, God was speaking through His prophet, Isaiah telling the people of Israel that He was there for them. That He was the help for Israel. Just like God was speaking to the nation of Israel, He is speaking those same words to you and to me. We don't need to be afraid (or fear), we don't need to be discouraged (or disappointed) because He is our God. He will strengthen and help us. And it is Him who will hold us up as we accomplish what He has for our lives.

Discouragement, from the Oxford dictionary, is defined as: 1) a loss of confidence or enthusiasm; or 2) an attempt to prevent something by showing disapproval or creating difficulties. Can you see how our disappointment in our circumstances can lead to fear and in turn discouragement? When we are disappointed in our situation, we can lose confidence in ourselves or in what our future may hold and because of that, our enthusiasm may seem to fade away too. We can convince ourselves that we can't do something, making it more difficult for us to accomplish the goals that we had previously set before us. Disappointment, fear and discouragement work together, trying to keep us from reaching our God given potential in our lives.

A cancer diagnosis doesn't mean that you can't accomplish the goals and ambitions that you have for yourself. Sure, it may delay them for a time but that doesn't mean that they can never be accomplished. We will talk about this a little later on, but we need to change our mindsets in these trying times in our lives. We need to stop allowing disappointment, fear and discouragement to control our thoughts, because when that happens those thoughts take action, or in most cases inaction, crippling us. Unfortunately, I understand how in moments like these it can be hard to take control over the thoughts and emotions that are clouding our lives, but we must do our best not to dwell on these things that cause nothing but worry and anxiety to an already stressful time in our lives.

I've always enjoyed looking back at the life of Joshua, and not just because he has a great name! Fun little fact, Joshua is the Old Testament name for Jesus, and means "Jehovah

(Jesus) Saves". Anyway, I have always liked Joshua because after Moses' death, when God appointed him to become the leader of the nation of Israel, he seemed to be a bit unsure of himself. I know that I have felt unsure about myself too, and it is nice to see a Biblical hero like Joshua experience those same feelings that I have in my life. Here was a man who was chosen by God to lead this group of rebellious Israelites into the Promised Land that they had been waiting to enter for generations. And I'm sure that throughout his time as Moses' assistant, seeing firsthand the attitude and actions of this group of people, he was probably overwhelmed with the responsibility that was given to him by God. Joshua was probably a bit disappointed that his mentor, Moses, was dead and would not be able to enter the Promised Land. He was sorely disappointed in the actions of the people he was now tasked to lead. There was probably fear of the uncertainty – would be able to lead the people the way that Moses did? Did he fear that they wouldn't listen to him or respect him? I'm sure that these things were very discouraging to Joshua at that time, and because of those feelings God spoke to Joshua.

Joshua 1:5-9 (NLT):

"No one will be able to stand against you as long as you live. For I will be with you as I was with Moses. I will not fail you or abandon you. Be strong and courageous, for you are the one who will lead these people to possess all the land I swore to their ancestors I would give them. Be strong and very courageous. Be careful to obey all the instructions Moses gave you. Do not deviate from them, turning either to the right or to the left. Then you will be successful in everything you do. Study this Book of Instruction continually. Meditate on it day and night so you will be sure to obey everything written in it. Only then will you prosper and succeed in all you do. This is

my command – be strong and courageous! Do not be afraid or discouraged. For the LORD your God is with you wherever you go."

Be strong and courageous. Did you catch that? Within five verses, God used that phrase to Joshua three different times, "Be strong and courageous." See the God who gave Joshua this enormous task, was also the One who was going to be with Joshua the entire time. He knew all of the disappointments Joshua had, all of the fears that were creeping into his mind and the discouragement that he was feeling. God wanted to let Joshua know that He was there in all of it. The LORD wasn't just telling Joshua to be strong and courageous so he could complete the job. No, He was showing Joshua that he could be strong and courageous because He was with him! How awesome is that?

Just like Joshua, the LORD is with us too. The last thing I want to point out is that if you continue to read the story of Joshua you will notice that those feelings followed him throughout his life's journey, and God would remind him again to be strong and courageous. Not only that, but Joshua repeated that same phrase multiple times when speaking to the nation of Israel. He told them, in turn reminding himself to be strong and courageous.

Just like Joshua and the nation of Israel, we too need to be reminded that God is with us. He is there in the hills and the valleys, the good times and the bad. He is ever present in our lives and is waiting on us to call out to Him. I can honestly say that without my relationship with God I don't know how I could have made it through those bouts of having cancer. I couldn't be strong enough or courageous enough on my own, no matter how hard I tried. It was only through Him that I was able to have the strength to carry on in those terrible times and find peace in my circumstance. So, I say to you, be strong and courageous, because God is with you.

CHAPTER 10

God In The Details

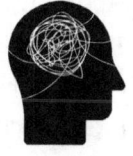

The older I get, the more I can look back at different times and moments in my life and see how God was with me. Too many times I go through each day not paying attention to God in the details of my life. I'm betting that you do too. My favorite verse in the Bible is Proverbs 16:33 (NLT):

"We may throw the dice, but the LORD determines how they fall."

It's such a simple verse, but has always spoken so powerfully to me, especially in those times I was going through cancer. In its simplicity it speaks so much truth. It doesn't matter what our plans are, how we think an outcome is going to take place, what we have studied, trained for or sacrificed for – God is ultimately in charge of the outcome. Do you think that as I was looking at what steps I needed to take in my life, how to position myself to succeed – in my marriage, my finances, my career path or any other part of my life– that I would have chosen to have cancer thrown into the mix? Absolutely not!

Let's see here...I'm going to finish up college, get married, land a great job, start a family, buy a house, and let's toss a year or two to halt all my plans to have cancer and forever change my life. Sounds like a solid plan, right? Let's be honest, no one thinks like that. We may plan for some hard times, but no one wants them or even really thinks that they will happen. Our dice have been thrown and we expect where we want them to land, but that's not always the case. God may have other plans for us and those plans may have cancer in them. But just because our dice don't land the way we want or expect doesn't mean that God isn't there.

For me it is important to look back on my life and see the blessings and miracles that God provided in the details of those moments in my life. It helps me to be encouraged that if He was with me before, He will continue to be with men now and in the future. When I see those God moments in my life it makes me so thankful that He cares for me and loves me enough to do special things in my life. Because of that I want to take some time to share a few different times throughout my cancer story that God was in the details of mine and Jamie's lives. My hope is that as you see how God was actively working in our lives, and that you will be encouraged to see how He is actively working in yours.

- It wasn't too long after I had finished chemo treatments, the first time I had cancer, when we got confirmation that we had made the right decision in not opting for the lymphadectomy (lymph node removal surgery). One day, while at work, my stepmother met a man who was having a hard time walking because one of his legs was abnormally larger than the other. It was apparently obvious that his condition was a recent issue for him and during their business interaction the subject of his leg came up. He told my stepmother that he had a lymphadectomy (the same surgery I was suggested by my first urologist). His leg issues were a side effect from that surgery. Thankfully, he didn't have any other issues, but that was bad enough. The reason his leg was so much larger than normal was because lymph node removal sometimes blocks drainage. You mainly see this swelling in the patient's arm or chest, called lymphedema. But in this man's case it was his leg that was building up fluid. This was because the excess fluid, which normally flows back into your bloodstream through the lymph system, was blocked due to the removal of his lymph nodes. I am terribly sorry that man had to deal with this issue, but after hearing of his story assured Jamie and myself that not doing that surgery was the correct choice for me.

- I have mentioned this previously, but I want to reiterate what a blessing my oncologist was. How there was confirmation that this doctor was the right decision for my care. After hearing about the not previously discussed option of chemotherapy from my first urologist, I had an appointment with the doctor who ended up becoming my oncologist and primary cancer treatment physician. My wife was unable to attend the initial doctor's visit to discuss the option of chemo, so my mother went with me for support and an extra set of ears, an extra mind and mouth for questions. From the moment that the doctor entered the room, both my mother and I had a sense of peace about her and about my treatment plan. As she began to talk to us about my cancer and her ideas for treatment, that peace grew even more. In only what I call "God-timing", she told us that she had just gotten back from a conference on testicular cancer. It was at that conference that the ineffectiveness of lymph node removal surgery being ineffective in the treatment of testicular cancer was discussed. Not only that, but one of her areas of expertise was, you guessed it, testicular cancer. Yet another confirmation that this is where God was leading me in my treatment.

- One thing about chemotherapy is that it comes in many "packages" to choose from, some short, some long, some larger dosages, some smaller ones. It can come in the form of a pill or liquid. You may have to do it for days or it could be years. Well, you get the point – there's a lot of different dosages, methods and timelines that can be used. What was an unexpected blessing was that because of the type of cancer that

I had, my age and my overall good health, minus the cancer, I was able to take a very large dose for a short amount of time. This was a blessing for a few different reasons mainly because it meant that I wouldn't be doing this for months or years. The faster you are done with chemo the better it is for your body and a less likely chance of a reappearance of new cancer growth. Small blessings in a hard time.

- For many years I have worn a rubber band around my left wrist. I started doing this so I could be reminded to pray about certain things. I often wrote down things that I was praying about onto my rubber band. During my second time having cancer, Jamie and I had a lot going on. She was pregnant with our son, Jonathan. We were in the process of moving into our first house. And...I had cancer for the second time. As many of you know none of those things are cheap and we hadn't finished financially recovering from the bills from the first bout with cancer. One of the things that I had written on my rubber band was "money". I can't even remember all of the ways that God has blessed us financially, but this one in particular was special. It was Christmastime and my mom and stepfather came over to our new house and brought some gifts, but these gifts weren't from them, they were from their coworkers. My mother and stepfather worked for the same company, a large grocery supplier and every year their office would adopt a family in need. Well when they announced the family that they would be adopting that year it was a surprise to my mom and stepdad too. They had decided, without either of them knowing, that they wanted to adopt Jamie and me because they knew that I was going through my second time with cancer. Like I said, they worked at a large grocery supplier and the employees would buy random items in bulk that would go to the adopted family. So the gifts were "odd" by Christmas standards, but we received cases of toilet paper and facial tissue just to name a few. It was pretty funny and we used all of the items over a long period of time. Blessings because we saved all kinds of money for the next year on odds and ends that you use around your house daily. The big "at the moment" need came when my mom handed me a Christmas box that was designed to look like a post office and you could open the top of the box that looks like the roof of the building. Inside of the box was a large sum of cash that their coworkers had pitched in to give to us. My prayers for money were answered. It wasn't a life-changing amount of money, but it was what we needed at the time, and we were so thankful. I remember telling my mom that I was going to put that post office box up every Christmas to remind me of that blessing, and I have done just that. Every year when we put up our Christmas decorations I am reminded of when God answered that prayer for money. And every year, I tell my son the same story of how God provided our financial need that Christmas. And every year he tells me "I know Dad, you tell me this every year." I just look at him and say it's good to remember when God answers your prayers and provides for you because you can be assured that He will do it again.

- When we had to cryogenically freeze my semen in case I became infertile, it was a tough decision because of the cost involved. It is a fairly pricey thing to do and we were a bit unsure if we could afford the cost at the time. Seeing a social worker was required by my oncologist's practice and the guy that I had to see found a program that drastically reduced the price, set up and storage of my specimen for a certain amount of time. I don't remember all of the details of the cost and everything associated with it, but through that program the costs basically only amounted to a couple of hundred dollars, which was a far cry away from what the price would have been without it. The assistance program was a huge financial blessing to us.

- One of the difficult things about my particular chemotherapy treatments was the fact that it knocked me down. During my treatments I was unable to do much at all other than lay around on the couch and feel miserable. It was such a chore to get up and walk to the bathroom, and Jamie would have to bathe me. Because of this I was unable to continue to work during my treatments and even for a couple of months after they were done. I also was unable to work after my surgery, because I was unable to lift, bend, stoop and walk very much for the first couple of weeks afterwards. Because of the surgery, chemotherapy and recovery/isolation period I ended up missing about three months of work both times that I had cancer. The huge God-sized blessing is that both times that I had cancer my companies paid my full salary the entire time I was out. They told me not to worry about short-term disability that they would pay me for whatever time that I needed to be out. How amazing is that? The really awesome thing is that I worked for a different company the second time that I had cancer, so two different companies decided that they would pay me my entire salary without having to use short term disability, which would have been significantly less money.

- After my first-time having cancer, the economy started to go down and my wife and I both lost our jobs. We were both unemployed for a year, other than my part-time job at our church being the student pastor. So that was fun... One of the really fun parts was that we did not have any medical insurance, and because of my history of cancer, I was unable to get any individual insurance policies for myself at the time. It was really unnerving. I had to stop with all preventive screenings, blood work and doctors visits because we couldn't afford to pay those out of pocket. When I finally landed a job, typically you must be at a company for at least three months before they give you insurance. Not this time! I was given insurance after my first month with the company! It was a huge blessing because it wasn't too long afterwards that I found out that I had cancer for the second time.

- Financial struggles when dealing with illnesses are common, as many of you well know, especially when you are just starting off in life – in my early 20's and newly married. At the time my wife was working for a company that had fantastic insurance with great benefits for cancer. Little did we know how great those benefits would actually be. My first surgery and chemo treatments only cost me $100 out of pocket outside of my normal copays for my visits. She didn't work there too long, honestly just a little before and a little after my first time having cancer but looking back we can now see why God led her to that job for that small season in our lives.

- One of the things that I believe can be overlooked in these chaotic times in our lives are some of the "smaller" blessings. Blessings that we may not notice at the time, but looking back are so important in those seasons. Some of those "small" blessings to me were my doctors. All of my doctors, except for my first urologist, specialized in my particular type of cancer. Testicular cancer isn't necessarily uncommon, but it's not as common as other types of cancers out there. God lead us to specialists in my area of need. Remember, my oncologist specialized in testicular cancer and had just gotten back from a meeting about it right before my first visit with her. I didn't even look her up, my first urologist office as a matter of convenience gave her name to me because her office was next to his and she worked within the same hospital group. My wife found my second urologist because his specialty was reproductive care with testicular cancer being a main study of his. The crazy thing about finding him was that my wife was looking through a totally different hospital group of doctors and somehow his name popped up. Coincidence? I think not. Then there was my pulmonologist, who did not need to specialize in cancer, but was a fantastic doctor. She was the doctor that doctors would see. She really was good in her field.

- After my second urologist told me that I needed to be on testosterone and to see an endocrinologist, we had to find one, and that was tough. Endocrinologists are very specialized doctors and have a decent number of patients. Because of that, it can take up to six months just to be seen. Well God was in this too. My wife was searching and found one who was accepting new patients and I was seen within the month. He was such a great guy, he was 80-years-old and only worked 3 days a week, but I was able to see him until he completely retired a couple of years later. His son was also an endocrinologist and after his dad retired, took me on as his patient with no lapse in my care. Both were great doctors and great men of God.

- More of those "small" maybe overlooked blessings that happened were the many people who prayed, visited and brought food over after my surgery and during my treatments. Receiving the food was a huge blessing to my wife, because it gave her a break from making food after working all day and taking care of me when she got off work. I also know that we can sometimes overlook those types of blessings because we typically don't see them as a big deal, but if you have received hospitality like that you know what a special thing it truly is.

- I had mentioned that during my second bout with cancer, we had just bought a house and my wife was pregnant. I had not started my chemotherapy treatments yet, but had just had my surgery and was still not supposed to be lifting anything heavier than a gallon of milk or doing much physical activity that could strain my incision site. Jamie, being pregnant, wasn't much better off than I was at the time and was unable to lift anything or do much manual labor either. Our house needed a few large projects done before we were able to move into it. Major cleaning, major painting and some general labor. We obviously were not able to do much of that, but our family, friends and church family stepped right in and took care of all of those things for us. Not only did they rescue us in the pre-move-in house preparation, but with our move as well. One of the men at the church owned a truck body shop and was able to use one of his trucks to load up all our stuff from our apartment and take it to our new house. On top of that we had a small army of folks show up to help from boxing up our things, to hauling them down four flights of stairs, loading them onto the truck, following us to our new house, unloading and helping set up our furniture. I can't tell you how thankful we were for all their help; we truly wouldn't have been able to do it without them.

• Our time was about to expire on our cryogenic storage, and we had to decide whether or not to keep my specimen, which was going to result in more payments, or to not renew our storage agreement and let them destroy my semen. I had several tests to see if my semen was viable and they all came back good. With that information we decided against renewing our storage agreement and had my specimen destroyed. Never thinking that I would ever have testicular cancer a second time, because there was only a 1% chance, we thought we were in the clear. It was right after the specimen was destroyed that Jamie became pregnant and not long after that I found out that I had testicular cancer for the second time. We had just been for Jamie's ultrasound to find out that we were having a boy. We were so excited! But our excitement was interrupted about 20 minutes after we found out by a phone call telling me the last semen test that I had taken showed that they were no longer viable. After we started to look back at the timing, when Jonathan was conceived, we realized how much of a miracle God had done in our lives. From the time that we decided to let the lab destroy my specimen, Jamie getting pregnant and me getting cancer the second time – making me infertile – there was only a one-month window in which Jamie could have gotten pregnant and we had been trying well before that month. What a miracle from God!

• The last miracle that I will tell you about is Jonathan. He truly is a miracle! Like I just told you about, Jamie and I had been trying to get pregnant with no luck for some time. After we decided to dispose of my specimen from the cryogenic lab, Jamie became pregnant and after the ultrasound where we found out we would be having a little boy I found out I could no longer have children of my own. We only had a month window for

Jamie to become pregnant, and we were unaware of this at the time of conception, but God knew. His hand was on our situation even when we were completely unaware of what was to come. He allowed Jamie to become pregnant at that specific time, knowing of the news we would soon receive. I can't thank Him enough for that blessing! Everyone we knew called Jonathan a miracle baby, because he was. We believe that names are special and important to God, because of how important names are throughout the Bible – even to the point where God changed people's names to reflect who He wanted them to be. Because of this, we named our son Jonathan, meaning God's Gift.

I know this isn't a complete list of all of the awesome things God did for us during this time of our lives, but I hope that you can see that even in the midst of what was a horrible time in our lives, God was with us. He was always there, even when we didn't know it at the time. I'm not anything special. Honestly, I have no idea why God chose to do all those wonderful blessings and miracles in my life, but He did. One thing I do know – because He did it for me, He can and will do the same for you.

I encourage you to look back at different times in your life and see how God moved in those moments. Reflect on those things and let them be an encouragement that He will continue to be with you today. Even when we may not be aware, He is there – loving, leading and guiding our way.

CHAPTER 11

Closing Thoughts

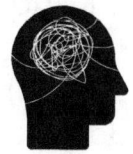

As we conclude our time together, I would like to thank you for listening to my story. I hope that my candidness about my cancer journey may have helped you see that you are not alone in your thoughts, feelings and emotions when it comes to your own cancer story. As you have heard me say many times already, I understand that not everyone's cancer experiences are like my own, some not as bad while many others are much worse. Even still, I believe that we can learn and even be encouraged by each other's testimonies of how we are dealing with or have dealt with our individual cancer experiences.

Hopefully as you have listened to my feelings, emotions and struggles throughout my experience, you can be encouraged to share your own experiences with others too. I believe it is important for others to hear our stories. People can relate and sympathize, while they are going through it. It is important for them to know that what they may be feeling isn't something that someone else hasn't had to deal with and overcome too. In all areas of my life, knowing that someone else has been where I am and has overcome some of the same obstacles that I may be facing, is comforting to me.

If you currently have cancer, remember, cancer doesn't automatically mean death. I understand that our modern culture and society seem to push those thoughts into our minds, but that is not true. Don't listen to the narrative that the world tells you, cancer doesn't have to be the end, rather it can be the beginning to a new chapter in the book of your life. This time will pass, just like so many other times in your life and you will eventually look back at it as something in the past, something that you overcame. I know that your present circumstances can be burdensome and it may be hard right now to look forward to the future, but know that this too will pass. Yes, it may always be in the background, just like it is with me, but trust me it's not always going to be like it is right now. I know it may be hard to believe now, but one day you too can look back at this time of your life and be thankful for it. There is that old saying that was even turned into a song, "What doesn't kill us, makes us stronger," and I believe that is true, especially in my own cancer journey. Something I would never have chosen for myself, has actually helped me grow, mature and see things in my life, with a whole new perspective – and I am grateful for it. You can be too.

I wish that all cancers didn't mean certain death but unfortunately there are some that are terminal. If you are facing terminal cancer, even though we may have never met, please know that I will be praying for you and your families. I also encourage whoever is reading this to do the same. You are experiencing thoughts and emotions I cannot speak on, but I do want to encourage you that even in this time of uncertainty in your life, God is still with you and will be with you throughout it all. Cry out to Him, pour yourself out to Him and let your heart be opened to receive what He has for you right now. Love your family and friends, and enjoy the time you have together.

I know a man who recently passed from this life to an eternity with Jesus, who was diagnosed with terminal brain cancer. At the time of his diagnosis he was given about two years to live and that timetable was accurate. I tell you this because, whereas this man was a Believer in Jesus Christ before his diagnosis, after he received the news it drew him closer to God than ever before. It was like he had a renewed passion to share the Gospel with others. He knew that his time here on earth was fading and he wanted to make the most of it before it was gone, and he did. He could have easily gotten very discouraged. I'm not saying that there weren't those times, but he didn't let those times dictate his final days. Because of that, he lived a very joyful last couple of years in his life here on earth. You too can have that as well. Even though I cannot relate to what you are going through personally, I have seen people dealing with similar situations who live thriving lives in spite of their diagnosis. I am encouraged that you too can and will thrive with the time that you have left.

To the person who may be reading this, who is supporting someone with cancer, thank you. You don't realize how much your love and support mean to the person who is dealing with a life-changing circumstance. I hope that you have been able to see my experience and better able to understand what your loved one is going though. Just because they may not seem outwardly upset about their situation doesn't mean that they are not dealing with many difficult thoughts and emotions. Encourage them, support them, help them and pray for them. I know that it may be hard dealing with them, just like my wife said that I was a horrible individual. I'm sure your loved one can be too. It's easier to be nice to people who aren't as close to you, but the ones you are really close with see the real you, the unfiltered you. We feel more comfortable to express our frustrations, emotions and pain and it may not come off too nice sometimes (or most of the time). Be patient with them, because they probably don't even realize that they are being rude or mean. Tell them in a loving way that they are not being nice or if you're my wife just tell them they are being a complete jerk. It's completely all right if you get frustrated too. It doesn't make you a bad person. You're dealing with this diagnosis too. I just encourage you to keep being supportive and to keep loving them even if they aren't deserving of it at the moment. I know it may not feel like it, but you are one of those blessings of God to the person you are supporting — keep up the good work!

If you are reading this just to see what all this cancer stuff is about and are not currently dealing with cancer in some way, thank you. Hopefully you never have to deal with cancer personally or even know or support someone that does, but the reality is that at some point, on some level, you will. Cancer is more prevalent now than ever and is expected to continue to become a bigger issue in the future. I'm grateful that you have chosen to expose and educate yourself on a topic that can be so uncomfortable. This is my personal testimony of my cancer story and everyone who has cancer will have a different story of his or her own. I am grateful that you decided to read this, and maybe one day you can be a blessing to someone who has cancer too.

Lastly, throughout my story I hope that you can see that the only way that I was able to endure this time of my life was because of my relationship with Jesus. You may remember me saying that I don't know how people handle a cancer diagnosis without a relationship with Jesus and I truly mean that. I'm unsure how I would have been able to handle going through those times without my faith in Him. I understand that if you are not a Christian some of the things that I have talked about may have been a bit uncomfortable for you, but I'm glad that you stuck around to the end anyway. You may be wondering how I got in this "relationship" with Jesus. So, before I close, I want to take a moment to share with you how you can have a relationship with Jesus in case you are the one who is wondering.

The Apostle Paul in the book of Romans spells it out pretty simply in these verses:

Romans 3:23 - *"For everyone has sinned; we all fall short of God's glorious standard."*

Romans 5:8 - *"But God showed his great love for us by sending Christ to die for us while we were still sinners."*

Romans 6:23 - *"For the wages of sin is death, but the free gift of God is eternal life through Christ Jesus our Lord."*

Romans 10:9-10 - *"If you openly declare the Jesus is Lord and believe in your heart that God raised him from the dead, you will be saved. For it is by believing in your heart that you are made right with God, and it is by openly declaring your faith that you are saved."*

Romans 10:13 – *"For everyone who calls on the name of the LORD will be saved."*

As we look over these scriptures we can see that all of us are sinners and fall short of God's standard and because of that He sent Christ to die for our sins. It is because of our sin that we will die, but we can have eternal life through Jesus Christ. All we have to do to receive His free gift of eternal life is confess that Jesus is Lord and believe that He was raised from the dead. When you do this you have entered into a relationship with Jesus and are "saved" (meaning you are saved from an eternal separation from God and you will have eternal life with God upon your death). It isn't some special prayer or magic words that "save" you, it is when you believe in your heart that you are made right with God, and by confessing your faith in Him that you are saved. It's not complicated; all you have to do is say a simple prayer something like this:

"Jesus I know that I am a sinner and I ask you to forgive me for all of my sins that I have committed against you. I believe that you died on the cross for my sins. I believe that you rose from the dead to overcome my sins and I am declaring my faith in you right now. Thank you for your free gift of salvation, even though I don't deserve

it. I accept that gift right now. Thank you for saving me! Amen."

I hope that if you have never made the decision to accept Jesus Christ into your life that you will truly consider making that decision at some point very soon. No one is deserving of God's faithfulness, His love or His free gift of salvation, but anyone who calls upon His name will be saved! We are not promised tomorrow, cancer or not, so let's do our best to make the most out of today!

www.ingramcontent.com/pod-product-compliance
Lightning Source LLC
Chambersburg PA
CBHW060543130626
46553CB00002B/877